This report contains the collective views of an international group of experts and does not necessarily represent the decisions or the stated policy of the United Nations Environment Programme, the International Labour Organization or the World Health Organization.

Environmental Health Criteria 235

DERMAL ABSORPTION

First draft prepared by Drs Janet Kielhorn, Stephanie Melching-Kollmuß, and Inge Mangelsdorf, Fraunhofer Institute of Toxicology and Experimental Medicine, Hanover, Germany

Published under the joint sponsorship of the United Nations Environment Programme, the International Labour Organization and the World Health Organization, and produced within the framework of the Inter-Organization Programme for the Sound Management of Chemicals.

World Health Organization

The **International Programme on Chemical Safety (IPCS)**, established in 1980, is a joint venture of the United Nations Environment Programme (UNEP), the International Labour Organization (ILO) and the World Health Organization (WHO). The overall objectives of the IPCS are to establish the scientific basis for assessment of the risk to human health and the environment from exposure to chemicals, through international peer review processes, as a prerequisite for the promotion of chemical safety, and to provide technical assistance in strengthening national capacities for the sound management of chemicals.

The **Inter-Organization Programme for the Sound Management of Chemicals (IOMC)** was established in 1995 by UNEP, ILO, the Food and Agriculture Organization of the United Nations, WHO, the United Nations Industrial Development Organization, the United Nations Institute for Training and Research and the Organisation for Economic Co-operation and Development (Participating Organizations), following recommendations made by the 1992 UN Conference on Environment and Development to strengthen cooperation and increase coordination in the field of chemical safety. The purpose of the IOMC is to promote coordination of the policies and activities pursued by the Participating Organizations, jointly or separately, to achieve the sound management of chemicals in relation to human health and the environment.

WHO Library Cataloguing-in-Publication Data

Dermal absorption.

(Environmental health criteria ; 235)

1.Skin absorption. 2.Risk assessment. 3.Environmental exposure.
I.World Health Organization. II.International Programme on Chemical Safety.
III.Series.

ISBN 92 4 157235 3 (NLM classification: WR 102)
ISBN 978 92 4 157235 4
ISSN 0250-863X

This document was technically and linguistically edited by Marla Sheffer, Ottawa, Canada, and printed by Wissenchaftliche Verlagsgesellschaft mbH, Stuttgart, Germany.

CONTENTS

ENVIRONMENTAL HEALTH CRITERIA FOR DERMAL ABSORPTION

NOTE TO READERS OF THE CRITERIA MONOGRAPHS

Every effort has been made to present information in the criteria monographs as accurately as possible without unduly delaying their publication. In the interest of all users of the Environmental Health Criteria monographs, readers are requested to communicate any errors that may have occurred to the Director of the International Programme on Chemical Safety, World Health Organization, Geneva, Switzerland, in order that they may be included in corrigenda.

Environmental Health Criteria

PREAMBLE

Objectives

In 1973, the WHO Environmental Health Criteria Programme was initiated with the following objectives:

(i) to assess information on the relationship between exposure to environmental pollutants and human health, and to provide guidelines for setting exposure limits;
(ii) to identify new or potential pollutants;
(iii) to identify gaps in knowledge concerning the health effects of pollutants;
(iv) to promote the harmonization of toxicological and epidemiological methods in order to have internationally comparable results.

The first Environmental Health Criteria (EHC) monograph, on mercury, was published in 1976, and since that time an ever-increasing number of assessments of chemicals and of physical effects have been produced. In addition, many EHC monographs have been devoted to evaluating toxicological methodology, e.g. for genetic, neurotoxic, teratogenic, and nephrotoxic effects. Other publications have been concerned with epidemiological guidelines, evaluation of short-term tests for carcinogens, biomarkers, effects on the elderly, and so forth.

Since its inauguration, the EHC Programme has widened its scope, and the importance of environmental effects, in addition to health effects, has been increasingly emphasized in the total evaluation of chemicals.

The original impetus for the Programme came from World Health Assembly resolutions and the recommendations of the 1972 UN Conference on the Human Environment. Subsequently, the work became an integral part of the International Programme on Chemical Safety (IPCS), a cooperative programme of WHO, ILO, and UNEP. In this manner, with the strong support of the new partners, the importance of occupational health and environmental effects was fully recognized. The EHC monographs have become widely established, used, and recognized throughout the world.

The recommendations of the 1992 UN Conference on Environment and Development and the subsequent establishment of the Intergovernmental Forum on Chemical Safety with the priorities for action in the six programme areas of Chapter 19, Agenda 21, all lend further weight to the need for EHC assessments of the risks of chemicals.

Scope

Two different types of EHC documents are available: 1) on specific chemicals or groups of related chemicals; and 2) on risk assessment methodologies. The criteria monographs are intended to provide critical reviews on the effect on human health and the environment of chemicals and of combinations of chemicals and physical and biological agents and risk assessment methodologies. As such, they include and review studies that are of direct relevance for evaluations. However, they do not describe *every* study carried out. Worldwide data are used and are quoted from original studies, not from abstracts or reviews. Both published and unpublished reports are considered, and it is incumbent on the authors to assess all the articles cited in the references. Preference is always given to published data. Unpublished data are used only when relevant published data are absent or when they are pivotal to the risk assessment. A detailed policy statement is available that describes the procedures used for unpublished proprietary data so that this information can be used in the evaluation without compromising its confidential nature (WHO (1990) Revised Guidelines for the Preparation of Environmental Health Criteria Monographs. PCS/90.69, Geneva, World Health Organization).

In the evaluation of human health risks, sound human data, whenever available, are preferred to animal data. Animal and in vitro studies provide support and are used mainly to supply evidence missing from human studies. It is mandatory that research on human subjects is conducted in full accord with ethical principles, including the provisions of the Helsinki Declaration.

The EHC monographs are intended to assist national and international authorities in making risk assessments and subsequent risk management decisions and to update national and international authorities on risk assessment methodology.

Procedures

The order of procedures that result in the publication of an EHC monograph is shown in the flow chart on p. xiii. A designated staff member of IPCS, responsible for the scientific quality of the document, serves as Responsible Officer (RO). The IPCS Editor is responsible for layout and language. The first draft, prepared by consultants or, more usually, staff from an IPCS Participating Institution, is based on extensive literature searches from reference databases such as Medline and Toxline.

The draft document, when received by the RO, may require an initial review by a small panel of experts to determine its scientific quality and objectivity. Once the RO finds the document acceptable as a first draft, it is distributed, in its unedited form, to well over 100 EHC contact points throughout the world who are asked to comment on its completeness and accuracy and, where necessary, provide additional material. The contact points, usually designated by governments, may be Participating Institutions, IPCS Focal Points, or individual scientists known for their particular expertise. Generally, some four months are allowed before the comments are considered by the RO and author(s). A second draft incorporating comments received and approved by the Coordinator, IPCS, is then distributed to Task Group members, who carry out the peer review, at least six weeks before their meeting.

The Task Group members serve as individual scientists, not as representatives of any organization, government, or industry. Their function is to evaluate the accuracy, significance, and relevance of the information in the document and to assess the health and environmental risks from exposure to the chemical or chemicals in question. A summary and recommendations for further research and improved safety aspects are also required. The composition of the Task Group is dictated by the range of expertise required for the subject of the meeting and by the need for a balanced geographical distribution.

EHC PREPARATION FLOW CHART

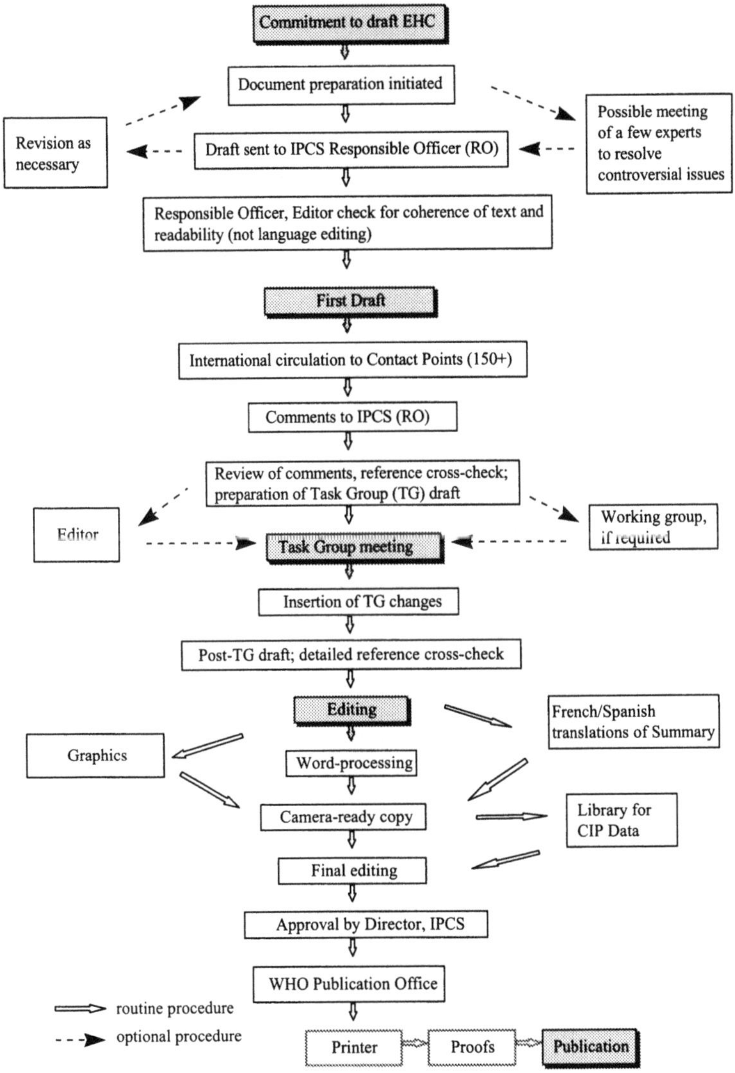

The three cooperating organizations of IPCS recognize the important role played by nongovernmental organizations. Representatives from relevant national and international associations may be invited to join the Task Group as observers. Although observers may provide a valuable contribution to the process, they can speak only at the invitation of the Chairperson. Observers do not participate in the final evaluation of the chemicals; this is the sole responsibility of the Task Group members. When the Task Group considers it to be appropriate, it may meet in camera.

All individuals who as authors, consultants, or advisers participate in the preparation of the EHC monograph must, in addition to serving in their personal capacity as scientists, inform the RO if at any time a conflict of interest, whether actual or potential, could be perceived in their work. They are required to sign a conflict of interest statement. Such a procedure ensures the transparency and probity of the process.

When the Task Group has completed its review and the RO is satisfied as to the scientific correctness and completeness of the document, it then goes for language editing, reference checking, and preparation of camera-ready copy. After approval by the Coordinator, IPCS, the monograph is submitted for printing.

It is accepted that the following criteria should initiate the updating of an EHC monograph: new data are available that would substantially change the evaluation; there is public concern for health or environmental effects of the agent because of greater exposure; an appreciable time period has elapsed since the last evaluation.

All Participating Institutions are informed, through the EHC progress report, of the authors and institutions proposed for the drafting of the documents. A comprehensive file of all comments received on drafts of each EHC monograph is maintained and is available on request. The Chairpersons of Task Groups are briefed before each meeting on their role and responsibility in ensuring that these rules are followed.

WHO TASK GROUP ON ENVIRONMENTAL HEALTH CRITERIA FOR DERMAL ABSORPTION

The first draft of the EHC monograph was prepared for IPCS by the Fraunhofer Institute, Hanover, Germany, in 2005. It was widely distributed by IPCS for international peer review for two months from March to May 2005. A revised proposed draft document, taking into account comments received, was prepared by the Fraunhofer Institute. An EHC Task Group was convened from 28 June to 1 July 2005, in Hanover, Germany, to further develop and finalize the document.

Ms C. Vickers was responsible for the production of the monograph.

The efforts of all who helped in the preparation and finalization of the monograph are gratefully acknowledged.

* * *

Risk assessment activities of IPCS are supported financially by the Department of Health and Department for Environment, Food & Rural Affairs, United Kingdom; Environmental Protection Agency, Food and Drug Administration, and National Institute of Environmental Health Sciences, USA; European Commission; German Federal Ministry of Environment, Nature Conservation and Nuclear Safety; Health Canada; Japanese Ministry of Health, Labour and Welfare; and Swiss Agency for Environment, Forests and Landscape.

Task Group Members

Dr R. Bronaugh, Office of Cosmetics and Colors, Food and Drug Administration, Laurel, MD, USA

Dr A.L. Bunge, Chemical Engineering Department, Colorado School of Mines, Golden, CO, USA

Dr J. Heylings, Central Toxicology Laboratory, Syngenta CTL, Alderley Park, Macclesfield, Cheshire, United Kingdom

Dr S. Kezic, Coronel Institute of Occupational and Environmental Health, Academic Medical Center, University of Amsterdam, Amsterdam, The Netherlands

Dr J. Krüse, Kinetox, Vleuten, The Netherlands

Dr U. Mueller, Office of Chemical Safety, Therapeutic Goods Administration, Woden, ACT, Australia

Dr M. Roberts, Department of Medicine, University of Queensland, Princess Alexandra Hospital, Buranda, Queensland, Australia (*Chairperson*)

Dr J.J.M. van de Sandt, Food and Chemical Risk Analysis, TNO Quality of Life, Zeist, The Netherlands

Dr K.A. Walters, Loughborough, United Kingdom

Professor F.M. Williams, Toxicology Unit and Environmental Medicine, The Medical School (School of Clinical Laboratory Sciences) and Institute for Research on Environment and Sustainability, University of Newcastle, Newcastle upon Tyne, United Kingdom

Secretariat

Dr J. Kielhorn, Department of Chemical Risk Assessment, Fraunhofer Institute of Toxicology and Experimental Medicine, Hanover, Germany (*Rapporteur*)

Dr I. Mangelsdorf, Department of Chemical Risk Assessment, Fraunhofer Institute of Toxicology and Experimental Medicine, Hanover, Germany

Dr S. Melching-Kollmuß, Department of Chemical Risk Assessment, Fraunhofer Institute of Toxicology and Experimental Medicine, Hanover, Germany

Ms C. Vickers, International Programme on Chemical Safety, World Health Organization, Geneva, Switzerland

ACRONYMS AND ABBREVIATIONS

ACGIH	American Conference of Governmental Industrial Hygienists
ADME	absorption, distribution, metabolism, and excretion
AOEL	acceptable operator exposure level
AUC	area under the curve
CEFIC	European Chemical Industry Council
CEFIC-LRI	European Chemical Industry Council Long-range Research Initiative
COLIPA	European Cosmetic Toiletry and Perfumery Association
DECOS	Dutch Expert Committee on Occupational Standards
DOEL	dermal occupational exposure limit
DPK	dermatopharmacokinetics
EC	European Commission
ECETOC	European Centre for Ecotoxicology & Toxicology of Chemicals
ECVAM	European Centre for the Validation of Alternative Methods
EDETOX	Evaluations and Predictions of Dermal Absorption of Toxic Chemicals
EHC	Environmental Health Criteria
EU	European Union
EURO POEM	European Predictive Operator Exposure Model
GC	gas chromatography
HPLC	high-performance liquid chromatography
ILO	International Labour Organization
IPCS	International Programme on Chemical Safety

J_{ss}	steady-state flux
K_m	vehicle/stratum corneum partition coefficient
K_{ow}	octanol/water partition coefficient
K_p	permeability coefficient
LC-MS	liquid chromatography/mass spectrometry
LD_{50}	median lethal dose
MAK	maximum allowable concentration (Germany)
MAK Commission	Senate Commission on the Investigation of Health Hazards of Chemical Compounds in the Work Area (Germany)
MW	molecular weight
NOAEL	no-observed-adverse-effect level
OECD	Organisation for Economic Co-operation and Development
OEL	occupational exposure limit
OSHA	Occupational Safety and Health Administration (USA)
PAH	polycyclic aromatic hydrocarbon
PPP	Perspectives in Percutaneous Penetration (formerly Prediction of Percutaneous Penetration)
QSAR	quantitative structure–activity relationship
QSPeR	quantitative structure–permeability relationship (also called QSPR)
REACH	Registration, Evaluation, Authorisation and Restriction of Chemicals
RO	Responsible Officer
SCCNFP	Scientific Committee on Cosmetic Products and Non-Food Products Intended for Consumers
SCOEL	Scientific Committee for Occupational Exposure Limits (European Union)
TLV	threshold limit value

TSCA	Toxic Substances Control Act (USA)
TWA	time-weighted average
UN	United Nations
UNEP	United Nations Environment Programme
USA	United States of America
USEPA	United States Environmental Protection Agency
USFDA	United States Food and Drug Administration
UV	ultraviolet
WHO	World Health Organization

1. SUMMARY

Dermal (percutaneous, skin) absorption is a global term that describes the transport of chemicals from the outer surface of the skin both into the skin and into the systemic circulation. This Environmental Health Criteria document presents an overview of dermal absorption and its application to the risk assessment of chemicals. In addition, it presents and discusses current topics of interest in the field of dermal absorption. Dermal absorption can occur from occupational, environmental, or consumer skin exposure to chemicals, cosmetics, and pharmaceutical products.

The skin is a complex organ and a living membrane. The functions of the skin include protection, regulation of body temperature and water loss, and defence and repair. The skin is composed of an outer region, the epidermis, and an inner region, the dermis. The epidermis consists of various cell layers, the outermost layer, the stratum corneum or horny layer, functioning as the main barrier to the entry of extraneous chemicals. The viable epidermis can metabolize chemicals that pass through the stratum corneum. The dermis provides physiological support for the avascular epidermis and is the locus of blood vessels, sensory nerves, and lymphatics in the skin. The skin also contains appendages, such as hair follicles, sweat glands, and sebaceous glands, which originate in the subpapillary dermis.

There is considerable variability in the measurement of skin permeability. There can be major differences in permeability between species. Little is known about variation due to age, although the skin structure does change with age; however, sex and ethnic background do not seem to be sources of variation in permeability. Percutaneous absorption is also dependent on the anatomical site, on the skin condition, and on the hydration state of the skin.

Factors influencing percutaneous absorption through the skin include 1) physicochemical properties of the test compound, 2) physicochemical and other properties of the vehicle in which the test compound is dissolved, 3) interactions between the test compound or vehicle and the skin, 4) skin properties and metabolism, and 5) factors inherent to the test system used for measurement — for example, dose and volume of test substance, occlusion or non-occlusion of test area, in vitro or in vivo test systems, and duration of exposure.

Theoretical equations and models have been developed to describe the transport of a diffusing chemical through the skin. Typically, the steady-state flux (J_{ss}) and the permeability coefficient (K_p) are the main parameters assessed from in vitro experiments in which the donor concentration of the penetrant is maintained at constant (infinite) dose conditions. The estimation of maximum flux, time for maximum flux, lag time, residual (reservoir) amounts retained in the stratum corneum, and mass balance under "real" application conditions is now recognized to be of prime importance in exposure estimations.

Measurement of metabolism of a chemical in contact with skin may be important in both efficacy and safety evaluations. Some chemicals can be significantly metabolized during dermal absorption, which may result in either inactive or active metabolites. The measurement of this metabolism may therefore be important in an appropriate safety evaluation. Toxic chemicals such as benzo[*a*]pyrene have been shown to be activated in skin, whereas other chemicals may undergo hydrolysis and/or conjugation reactions in the skin, resulting in a decrease in the availability of those chemicals to the body. In general, the viability of skin can be maintained in an in vitro diffusion cell by using fresh skin and a physiological buffer. It is recommended that this viability be verified through measuring the activity of relevant metabolizing enzymes.

The permeability properties of the stratum corneum are, for the most part, unchanged after its removal from the body. As a consequence, a good correlation exists between measurements derived from both in vivo and in vitro skin diffusion experiments with the same chemicals (at least for hydrophilic compounds). In vitro experiments are an appropriate surrogate for in vivo studies and offer a number of advantages over whole-animal or human volunteer experiments. In vitro methods measure the diffusion of chemicals into and across skin to a fluid reservoir and can utilize non-viable skin to measure diffusion only or fresh, metabolically active skin to simultaneously measure diffusion and skin metabolism. Test Guideline 428 of the Organisation for Economic Co-operation and Development (OECD) encourages harmonization of methodology. Experimental factors affecting dermal absorption in vitro, in addition to those mentioned above, include the thickness of skin sample, variations in temperature of the test system, and composition of the receptor fluid. Static or flow-through in vitro diffusion cells can be used. Additional techniques, requiring further refinements, include tape stripping and the use of artificial or reconstituted skin.

In vivo methods allow the determination of the extent of cutaneous uptake as well as systemic absorption of the test substance. The main advantage of performing an in vivo study rather than an in vitro study is that it uses a physiologically and metabolically intact system. In vivo dermal penetration studies are carried out in laboratory animals, usually rodents, and in human volunteers. In vivo dermal penetration studies in human volunteers have been widely used for human pharmaceuticals and, to a more limited extent, for other chemicals. In vivo studies in humans are the gold standard. The conduct of any in vivo study has ethical issues. The main disadvantage in the use of laboratory animals is that they have different skin permeability and systemic disposition compared with humans.

The results of human volunteer studies have shown that occupational exposure to liquids (such as solvents) can result in considerable dermal absorption. Skin uptake from vapours may be an important contributor to the total uptake for some volatile substances, such as the glycol ethers.

In vitro dermal absorption studies are increasingly being submitted for registration purposes for industrial chemical, cosmetic, and crop protection products. There are many published studies that compare in vitro and in vivo results in laboratory animals and humans. Properly conducted in vitro studies that follow the OECD test guidelines have demonstrated that the in vitro approach can provide good prediction of in vivo dermal absorption.

Over the decades, a large number of data have been generated on the percutaneous penetration of a wide range of chemicals, pesticides, cosmetics, and pharmaceuticals. Studies have included work on human volunteers, in vivo studies using animal models, in vitro studies on excised human, rodent, pig, guinea-pig, etc., skin, and, more recently, in vitro studies on synthetic skin.

There have been many attempts over the last 50 years to predict the rate and extent of dermal absorption and so reduce the need for in vitro and in vivo testing. This need is even greater in response to increasing ethical difficulties with respect to human and laboratory animal experiments as well as the legislatively imposed economic and time considerations — particularly in the risk assessment of industrial chemicals. Quantitative structure–permeability relationships (QSPeRs) are statistically derived relationships between the steady-state flux of a compound and various physicochemical descriptors and/or structural properties of the molecule. Efficacy and safety considerations also recognize quantitative structure–activity relationships (QSARs) in irritation, skin sensitization, metabolism, chemical effects, and clearance. QSARs are therefore involved at a number of levels in chemical safety.

Mathematical models have been used to simulate the dynamics of the partition, diffusion, metabolism, and other processes involved in dermal absorption and can lead to the prediction of the extent and rate of chemical permeation through the skin. Mathematical modelling plays a key role in linking permeability coefficient and flux data obtained from tests under steady-state conditions (i.e. infinite dose) to absorption estimates for finite dose applications that are more typical of occupational exposure (i.e. non-steady-state conditions).

In risk assessment, the initial estimate for dermal absorption is usually obtained by the use of a tiered approach, where the greatest safety margin is defined by the worst case and more refined estimates better define the real margin. Hence, as a first step, 100% absorption is assumed when no data are available. In the second step, a more realistic estimate of the extent of dermal absorption is provided by a consideration of the physicochemical properties of the chemical and the vehicle. The third step is a consideration of any experimental in vitro and in vivo dermal absorption data. If, at the end of these steps, an unacceptable risk is calculated, the risk assessment is best refined by means of actual exposure data.

In the last few years, partly due to regulatory pressures, there have been several initiatives to accelerate progress in the fields of international harmonization of methodology and protocols, culminating in the publication of the OECD test guidelines for skin absorption studies in 2004. This international collaboration includes projects such as an international validation study involving 18 laboratories, the European Evaluations and Predictions of Dermal Absorption of Toxic Chemicals (EDETOX) project, and projects sponsored by industry, as well as conferences, such as the Perspectives in Percutaneous Penetration (formerly the Prediction of Percutaneous Penetration, or PPP) and Gordon Research conferences. Available data on skin fluxes and permeability coefficients have been collected into databases and analysed. Progress has been made in further developing QSARs that link permeation data to the physicochemical properties of chemicals. As a consequence, it is becoming increasingly possible to more reliably predict penetration data for a large number of chemicals. A possible outcome is a reduction in the expensive and ethically demanding testing of chemicals using laboratory animals and humans.

In spite of the successes in interdisciplinary international harmonization to date, there are a number of aspects to be further improved and which remain as topics of discussion. These include the extent of intralaboratory and interlaboratory variation in in vitro and in vivo studies; the acceptance of QSPeRs; the reservoir effect of chemicals in the stratum corneum and its interpretation in risk assessment; the relevance of dermal absorption measurements to data required by risk assessors; and the use of the barrier integrity test for skin barrier function. Other topics that must be considered include dermal absorption in susceptible populations, the necessity for harmonization of skin notation, and the dermal absorption of nanoparticles.

Recommendations are made by the Task Group concerning the benefits of using human skin over laboratory animal skin; study design and harmonization of methodology; correlation of in vitro and in vivo data and development of reliable prediction models; encouraging support, maintainance, and update of databases; and furthering the evaluation of QSARs for risk assessment purposes, and preparation of guidance on their use.

2. INTRODUCTION AND DEFINITIONS

2.1 Scope of the document

Chemicals present in workplaces or the environment may come into contact with the skin and be absorbed. Although interest in dermal absorption for risk assessment purposes is comparatively recent, research into the factors involved in the passage of compounds through the skin has been conducted for other purposes. Some scenarios where dermal absorption considerations are important include:

- the development of transdermal drug delivery systems (e.g. for analgesia);
- dermatological formulations for localized transport (e.g. psoriasis);
- safety assessment of cosmetics; and
- risk assessment of occupational, environmental, or consumer exposure.

Although these applications involve dermal absorption, they all have different aims and approaches. For some drugs, it may be important that the substance passes through the skin and into the bloodstream. For cosmetics and sunscreen lotions, it may not be necessary or desirable for the product to penetrate the skin; instead, the product may simply remain in the upper skin layer.

In occupational and consumer scenarios, the skin absorption of chemicals and pesticides needs to be minimized. Risk assessments are usually performed to determine the extent to which exposure to a particular substance is acceptable and therefore the extent to which the substance is safe to use. For many chemicals, there is no information on dermal absorption.

This Environmental Health Criteria document concentrates on dermal absorption from occupational, environmental, or consumer exposure, which may involve exposure to liquids, solids, or vapours. The exposure to liquids is usually intermittent; volatile substances may evaporate from the skin surface. Occupational exposure may be single or repeated, thus requiring risk assessment and control.

The steps between the presence of a chemical in the environment and systemic exposure may be divided into two phases (Johanson, 2003). The first phase is the dermal exposure to the chemical (amount, area, duration). This is affected by a number of factors, such as the properties of the chemical, the work process, the individual's behaviour and work practices, type of clothing, type of protective equipment, etc. This document does not cover these aspects. It deals with the second phase, that from exposure of the skin to systemic exposure — the dermal absorption.

The purpose of this document is to present to the newcomer an overview of dermal (percutaneous) absorption (chapters 3–5) and its measurement (chapters 6–8), in particular with regard to the risk assessment of chemicals. It does not intend to be comprehensive. A further aim is to present and discuss current topics of interest in the field of percutaneous penetration. In the last few years, partly due to regulatory pressures, there have been several initiatives to accelerate progress in the fields of international harmonization of methodology and protocols, culminating in the publication of the Organisation for Economic Co-operation and Development (OECD) test guidelines for skin absorption studies in 2004 (OECD, 2004a,b,c; see Appendix 1) and the European Evaluations and Predictions of Dermal Absorption of Toxic Chemicals (EDETOX) project (Appendix 2). Further, available data on permeation have been collected into databases (see chapter 9), and progress has been made in developing quantitative structure–activity relationships (QSARs) linking physicochemical properties to permeation data so that in the future it may be possible to predict the data for a large number of chemicals rather than undertake expensive testing of chemicals (see chapter 10 and Appendix 2). In addition, projects have been initiated to investigate risk assessment processes (chapter 11). In spite of these successes in interdisciplinary international harmonization, there are still points that are topics of discussion (chapter 12), and a way forward is proposed (chapter 13).

Owing to the large amount of literature available, only some specific studies are cited. In the respective chapters throughout the document, however, the reader is referred to reviews where more information can be found.

2.2 Definition of dermal absorption

Dermal (percutaneous, skin) absorption is a global term that describes the transport of chemicals from the outer surface of the skin to the systemic circulation (OECD, 2004a). This is often divided into:

- *penetration*, which is the entry of a substance into a particular layer or structure, such as the entrance of a compound into the stratum corneum;
- *permeation*, which is the penetration through one layer into a second layer that is both functionally and structurally different from the first layer; and
- *resorption*, which is the uptake of a substance into the skin lymph and local vascular system and in most cases will lead to entry into the systemic circulation (systemic absorption).

These definitions will be used in this document. However, it should be recognized that these terms may be interpreted differently in the various product sectors.

2.3 Factors influencing dermal absorption

There are a number of factors that influence the dermal absorption of a substance, and some of these are listed in Table 1. These and other factors are more fully discussed in the appropriate sections of the document.

Table 1. Some important considerations in dermal absorption

System components	Factors	Discussion in
Test compound	Physical state	Chapters 4 and 10
	Molecular size	
	Lipid/water partition coefficient	
	Ionization	
	Local skin effects	
Skin	Species	Chapters 3, 5, 6, and 7
	Anatomical site	
	Temperature	
	Hydration of stratum corneum	
	Damage to stratum corneum	
	Metabolism	
	Diseased skin	
	Desquamation	
	Blood and lymph flow	
Vehicle	Solubility	Chapters 6 and 7
	Volatility	
	Distribution in stratum corneum	
	Excipients	
	Effect on the stratum corneum	
	pH	
Application dose	Concentration	Chapters 6 and 7
	Finite and infinite dose	
	Skin area dose (film thickness, concentration)	
	Total skin area in contact with vehicle	
	Duration of exposure	
Other factors	Reservoir effect and its interpretation in risk assessment	Chapters 3, 6, and 12

3. SKIN STRUCTURE AND FUNCTION

The skin is the largest organ in the body, with a surface area of approximately 1.8 m^2 and a total weight estimated, for a typical adult of 70 kg, to be 4 kg (Pannatier et al., 1978). In normothermic conditions, the cutaneous circulation comprises 5–10% of the total cardiac output (Johnson et al., 1986). For 70-kg human males, the skin blood flow is approximately 4.64 cm^3/s or 16 700 cm^3/h (Kasting & Robinson, 1993). Thus, the ratio of the total capillary flow to the corresponding skin surface area is approximately 0.93 cm/h.

The skin is a heterogeneous organ, containing a number of layers as well as appendages, such as sweat glands, hair follicles, and sebaceous glands (see Figure 1). The thickness of the skin and composition of the stratum corneum vary according to body region. Until the beginning of the 20th century, the skin was thought to be completely inert and impermeable to chemicals that might otherwise enter the body. While the skin does act as a barrier, it is not a complete barrier. Many chemicals do penetrate the skin, either intentionally or unintentionally, and cutaneous metabolism does occur. Because of its large surface area, the skin may be a major route of entry into the body in some exposure situations.

Several authors have provided more extensive reviews of the topics addressed in this section (e.g. Wiechers, 1989; Singh & Singh, 1993; Schaefer & Redelmeier, 1996; Walters & Roberts, 2002; Madison, 2003; Monteiro-Riviere, 2004, 2005).

3.1 Functions of the skin

3.1.1 Barrier function

The skin provides a sturdy, flexible, and self-repairing barrier to the exterior environment, protecting the internal body organs and fluids from external influences. It prevents loss of endogenous water and nutrients (humans are approximately 70% water) and protects against many unwanted toxic substances and pathogenic microorganisms. The skin also responds to mechanical forces (elasticity and cushioning).

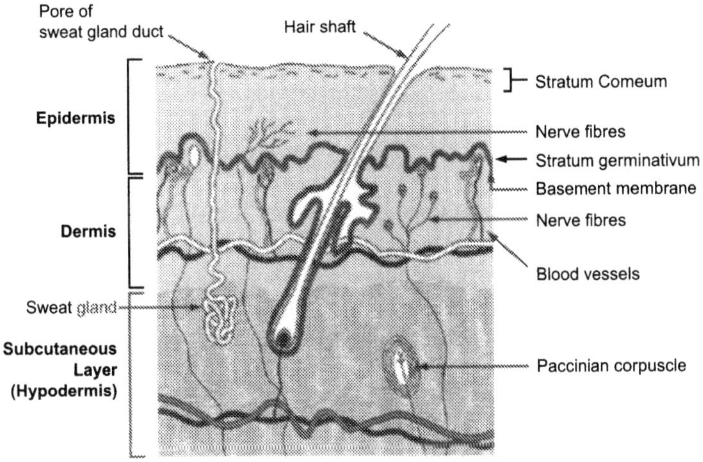

Fig. 1. A schematic diagram of the structure of the skin.

3.1.2 *Temperature control*

The skin plays an essential role in the control of body temperature, which is regulated by sweating and arteriovenous thermoregulation. The skin's resting blood flow of 250–300 cm^3/min can increase to 6000–8000 cm^3/min in response to an increase in internal body temperature, with much of the flow going directly from arterioles to venules (Cross & Roberts, 2005).

3.1.3 *Defence and repair*

The skin contains systems that provide the ability for defence and repair, such as touch sensitivity (Merkel cells, nociceptors), immunity (Langerhans cells), protection against ultraviolet (UV) radiation (melanocytes), wound healing, and cutaneous metabolism. Repair occurs automatically through the continuous turnover of the skin, but this mechanism can be accelerated via cytokine release following insult or injury.

3.2 Skin structure

Based on structure and embryonic origin, the cellular layers of the skin are divided into two distinct regions. The outer region, the *epidermis*, develops from the embryonic ectoderm and covers the connective tissue; the *dermis* is derived from the mesoderm (Maibach & Patrick, 2001; Monteiro-Riviere, 2005).

3.2.1 Epidermis

The epidermis comprises about 5% of full-thickness skin and is divided into five or six layers, based on cellular characteristics (see Figure 2). The majority of cells in the epidermis are called keratinocytes, which are formed by differentiation from one layer of mitotic basal cells. The number of distinguishable layers is dependent upon the anatomical site.

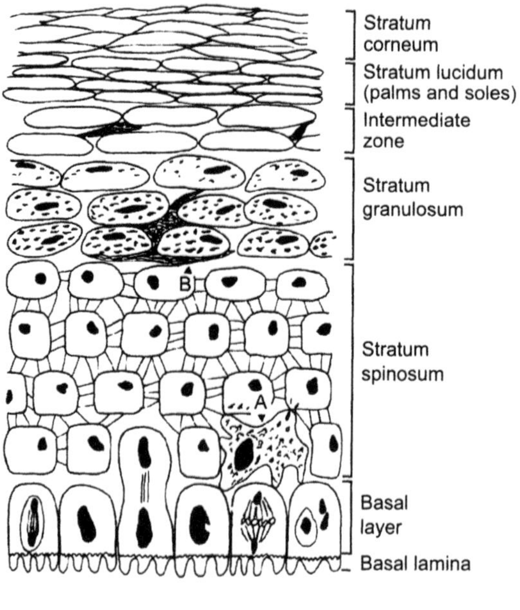

Fig. 2. The epidermis. All cell layers and locations of the two dendritic cell types, melanocytes (A) and Langerhans cells (B), are shown (Maibach & Patrick, 2001). [Copyright (2001) From Principles and Methods of Toxicology by W.A. Hayes. Reproduced by permission of Routledge/Taylor & Francis Group, LLC]

Basal layer (stratum germinativum) keratinocytes are metabolically active cells with the capacity to divide. Some of the resulting daughter cells of the basal layer move outward and differentiate. The cells adjacent to the basal layer start to produce lamellar granules, intracellular organelles that later fuse with the cell membrane to release the neutral lipids that are thought to form a barrier to penetration through the epidermis (see next paragraph). The desmosomes (adhesive junctions; Hatsell & Cowin, 2001) and other bridges connecting the adjacent cells have the appearance of spines, giving the name stratum spinosum to this three- to four-cell-thick layer above the basal layer. The keratinocytes migrate outwards to the third epidermal layer, called the stratum granulosum, which is characterized by the presence of keratohyalin granules, polyribosomes, large Golgi bodies, and rough endoplasmic reticulum. These are the outermost viable cells of the epidermis.

The major barrier to permeation within the skin is the non-viable stratum corneum, the outermost cornified layer, usually 15–20 cells thick and consisting of cells (corneocytes) that have lost their nucleus and all capacity for metabolic activity. The dominant constituent of these cells is keratin, a scleroprotein with chains linked by disulfide and hydrogen bonds. The corneocytes are connected by corneodesmosomes and surrounded by extracellular non-polar lipids. The stratum corneum intercellular barrier lipids originate in the lamellar granules most prominent in the granular cell layer of the epidermis (Madison, 2003). Each corneocyte is enclosed within a protein-rich cornified cell envelope that provides covalent linkage sites for the intercellular lipids.

The process of desquamation disrupts intercellular attachment, and the outermost cells are sloughed from the surface. The turnover rate for keratinocytes has been calculated to be between 17 and 71 days, depending upon anatomical site: e.g. 32–36 days for the human palm and 58 days for the anterior surface of the forearm (Maibach & Patrick, 2001). Although the thickness of non-hydrated stratum corneum is about 10–50 µm over most of the body, it may be 10 times thicker on friction surfaces such as the hands and soles of the feet (Rushmer et al., 1966), where the corneodesmosomes also have a higher prevalence than in other skin regions. The stratum corneum has a water content of 5–20%, compared with 70% in the physiologically active basal layer.

Owing to the relative impermeability of the cornified envelope to most compounds, the major route of penetration across the stratum corneum has been identified as the tortuous pathway between the corneocytes (see Figure 3), implying that stratum corneum lipids play a key role in the skin barrier function (Michaels et al., 1975; Elias, 1981; Grubauer et al., 1987; Mao-Qiang et al., 1993; Bouwstra et al., 2001, 2003a; Ponec et al., 2003).

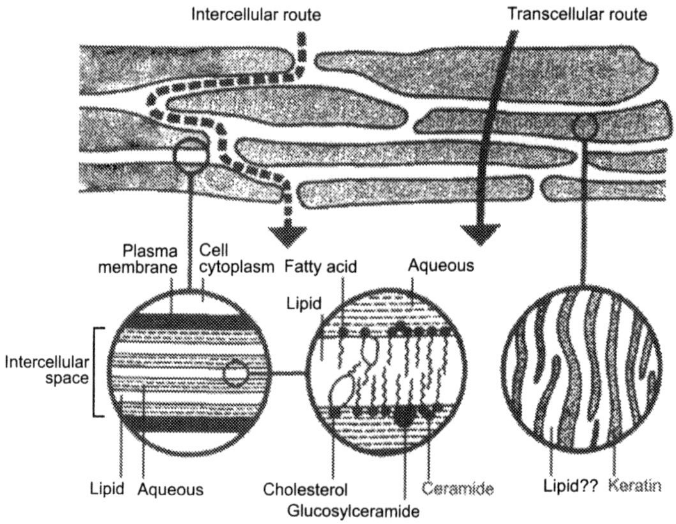

Fig. 3. Diagram of the stratum corneum membrane, showing two possible routes for diffusion (Barry, 1991). [Copyright (1991) From In Vitro Percutaneous Absorption: Principles, Fundamentals, and Applications by R.L. Bronaugh and H.I. Maibach. Reproduced by permission of Routledge/Taylor & Francis Group, LLC]

The hydrophobic lipids present in the intercellular spaces of the stratum corneum are (all weight per cent) 45–50% ceramides, 25% cholesterol, 15% long-chain free fatty acids (mostly with chain lengths C22 and C24), and 5% other lipids, the most important being cholesterol sulfate, cholesterol esters, and glucosylceramides (Wertz et al., 1987; Law et al., 1995; Madison, 2003). Nine subclasses of ceramides have been identified in human stratum corneum (de Jager et al., 2003; Ponec et al., 2003). The ceramides consist of a sphingosine or a phytosphingosine base to which a non-hydroxy fatty acid or an alpha-hydroxy fatty acid is chemically linked (see Figure 4). The fatty acid chain is mainly C24 and C26. Cholesterol sulfate, although present in only small amounts, has been shown to be involved in the regulation of the desquamation process. The importance of the relationship between lipid organization and composition has been shown from studies with diseased skin in which an impaired barrier function paralled altered lipid composition and organization (Bouwstra et al., 2001; Kalinin et al., 2002; Madison, 2003).

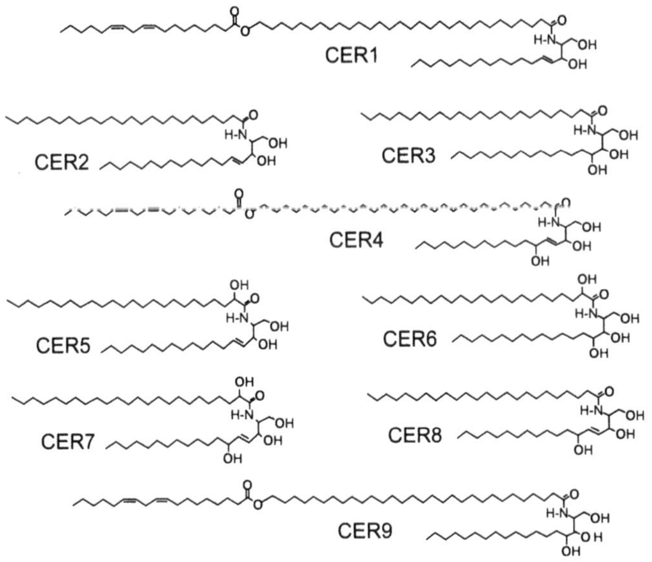

Fig. 4. Molecular structure of ceramides (CER) in human stratum corneum (de Jager et al., 2003). [Reprinted from Chemistry and Physics of Lipids, Vol. 124, No. 2, M.W. de Jager et al., The phase behaviour of skin lipid mixtures based on synthetic ceramides, pp. 123–134, Copyright (2003), with permission from Elsevier]

In addition to keratinocytes, the epidermis contains two dendritic cell types — melanocytes and Langerhans cells. Melanocytes lie directly adjacent to the basal layer and produce melanin, the principal pigment of human skin, which is then transferred to basal layer keratinocytes. Langerhans cells bear Ia (immune recognition) antigens and have surface receptors for the Fc portion of immunoglobulin G and 3b, a component of complement C3 (Ahmed, 1979; Romani et al., 2003). Langerhans cells lie in epidermal layers containing enzymes that can metabolize exogenous chemicals.

3.2.2 Dermis

The dermis provides the nutritional support for the avascular epidermis. The dermis is a 0.2- to 0.3-cm-thick tissue that comprises a fibrous protein matrix, mainly collagen, elastin, and reticulum, embedded in an amorphous colloidal ground substance. The physical behaviour of the dermis, including elasticity, is determined by the fibre bundles and ground substance. The dermis is the locus of blood vessels, sensory nerves (pressure, temperature, and pain), and lymphatics. It contains the inner segments of the sweat glands and pilosebaceous units. The dermis provides flexibility with strength, serves as a barrier to infection, and functions as a water storage organ (Singh & Singh, 1993).

3.2.3 Skin appendages

The skin appendages originate in the subpapillary dermis and consist of eccrine sweat glands, apocrine sweat glands, sebaceous glands, and hair follicles, with their associated erector muscles. Appendages are found in most anatomical sites, although the number of each varies significantly by site. An average human skin surface contains 40–70 hair follicles and 200–250 sweat ducts per square centimetre. Sebaceous glands are most numerous and largest on the face, especially the forehead, in the ear, on the midline of the back, and on anogenital surfaces. They secrete sebum, the principal components being glycerides, free fatty acids, cholesterol, cholesterol esters, wax esters, and squalene. Sebum acts as a skin lubricant and a source of stratum corneum plasticizing lipid and maintains acidic conditions (pH 5) on the skin's outer surface.

The eccrine glands are epidermal structures that are simple coiled tubes arising from a coiled ball of approximately 100 μm in diameter located in the lower dermis. These glands secrete a dilute salt solution with a pH of about 5. This secretion is stimulated by temperature-controlling determinants, such as exercise and high environmental temperature, as well as emotional stress, through the autonomic (sympathetic) nervous system. The apocrine glands are limited to specific body regions (e.g. armpit, the breast areola, and the perianal region) and are about 10 times larger than eccrine ducts. The apocrine glands, present after puberty, are sweat ducts in axillary skin.

3.3 The transport of chemicals through the skin

The transport of chemicals through the skin is a complex process. The skin is a complex organ and also a living membrane. The skin and the environment are in constant interaction.

There are three major mechanisms by which skin absorption may occur (see also Figures 1 and 3):

1) *Transcellular absorption*: The chemical is transferred through the keratin-packed corneocytes by partitioning into and out of the cell membrane.

2) *Intercellular absorption*: The chemical is transferred around the corneocytes in the lipid-rich extracellular regions.

3) *Appendageal absorption*: The chemical bypasses the corneocytes, entering the shunts provided by the hair follicles, sweat glands, and sebaceous glands.

As the relative surface area of these shunts (appendages) is only 0.1–1.0% of the total area, they are not thought to play a decisive role in the absorption of many chemicals in humans. However, the relative surface area of the shunts may be of greater significance in areas of the body such as the scalp, where the density and size of hair follicles are much greater than in, for example, the skin of the back. Further, these shunts may be important at early time points following application of the penetrant. Sebaceous glands may act as a drug reservoir for some materials (Scheuplein, 1967).

3.4 Variability in skin permeability

3.4.1 Species

There are significant differences between the dermal absorption observed in laboratory animals and that in humans (see also sections

6.5 and 7.4). For the majority of chemicals, laboratory animal skin is considerably more permeable (ECETOC, 1993; Vecchia & Bunge, 2005). Differences in the lipid content, structure, and thickness of the stratum corneum are important factors (Walters & Roberts, 1993). Laboratory animal skin has a much higher number of appendageal openings per unit surface area than human skin, and this may be an additional causative factor for compounds for which appendageal transport may be significant. The skin of weanling pigs and monkeys appears to be the most predictive model for human percutaneous penetration (Wester & Maibach, 1985; see also chapter 7).

A review of permeability coefficient data for several animal species (rats, mouse, snake, etc.) is provided by Vecchia & Bunge (2005).

3.4.2 Age, sex, and race

Premature and low-birth-weight babies have a poorly developed stratum corneum, but they develop a competent barrier within 4 weeks after birth (Kalia et al., 1996).

Changes that occur in ageing skin include 1) increased stratum corneum dryness, 2) reduction in sebaceous gland activity, resulting in a decrease in the amount of skin surface lipids, 3) flattening of the dermal–epidermal junction, and 4) atrophy of the skin capillary network, resulting in a gradual attenuation of blood supply to the viable epidermis. Some studies have shown that the barrier function of the skin increases with increasing chronological age and that relatively hydrophilic compounds are particularly sensitive. However, little is known about the influence of such age-related changes on percutaneous absorption (Roskos et al., 1989).

In general, regardless of environmental conditions, sex, and ethnic background, the barrier properties of the skin are reasonably similar. No observable differences were found in the percutaneous absorption of benzoic acid, caffeine, or acetylsalicylic acid between Asian, black, and Caucasian subjects (Lotte et al., 1993). However, it should be pointed out that all investigated compounds were hydrophilic.

3.4.3 Anatomical site

The skin thickness of the eyelid is approximately 0.05 cm and that of the palm and sole about 0.4 cm (Maibach & Patrick, 2001). Percutaneous absorption varies depending on the site of the body (Feldmann & Maibach, 1967; Wester & Maibach, 1999a; see also chapter 7). There is also considerable variability at a given site and within and between individuals (Southwell et al., 1984).

3.4.4 Skin condition

Skin condition can have a significant impact on the penetration and permeation of chemicals, especially when the barrier function is disrupted. The permeability of the skin can be increased by physical (e.g. weather, sunlight, occlusion), chemical (e.g. solvents, detergents, acids, alkalis), and pathological factors (e.g. mechanical damage, disease state) (Wiechers, 1989). Mixtures of polar and non-polar solvents delipidize the skin, resulting in a substantial reduction of the barrier function.

Some of the most common skin diseases, such as psoriasis and atopic eczema, are characterized by a virtual absence of the granular layer in the viable epidermis. In psoriasis, the proliferation is excessive, but keratinization is incomplete (Barry, 1983). There are several genetic skin diseases with known defects in lipid metabolism that have scaly or ichthyotic skin as part of the clinical picture (for details, see Williams & Elias, 2000; Madison, 2003). However, in diseased skin, the degree of barrier efficiency may vary widely and depends on the precise pathological state of the stratum corneum (see also section 12.7).

3.4.5 Temperature and blood flow rate

Skin temperature can have an impact on the rate of penetration of chemicals in two different ways (Bunge & McDougal, 1999). First, increasing the temperature of the skin has been shown to increase the rate of penetration by a direct effect on the diffusion within the skin (Scheuplein & Blank, 1971). Temperature can also affect the structure of the stratum corneum, particularly the crystalline structure of the lipid bilayers (Pilgram et al., 1999; de Jager et al., 2004), which can lead to higher permeability. Second, temperature may affect blood flow to the skin. However, this mainly affects the amount of lipophilic chemicals absorbed, as their clearance by the blood is often rate limiting (Cross & Roberts, 2005). Clearance into the blood is also dependent on the physiology of the skin. Warming the skin will increase cutaneous blood flow, and the penetration rate through the skin may increase, but some of the dermal blood is shunted through anastomoses to facilitate skin cooling. Such flow is less effective than nutritive dermal blood flow in clearing chemicals from the epidermis (Cross & Roberts, 2005). In general, blood clearance is of importance for small, moderately lipophilic chemicals that penetrate the skin rapidly but absorb into the blood slowly (Siddiqui et al., 1989).

3.4.6 *Hydration*

The stratum corneum normally contains 5–20% water, but it can contain up to 50% when hydrated, and this can affect the permeability of the skin to chemicals (Scheuplein & Blank, 1971; Roberts & Walker, 1993; Bouwstra et al., 2003b; Warner et al., 2003; Rawlings & Matts, 2005). Idson (1971) claimed that increasing hydration increases the absorption of all substances that penetrate the skin. However, increasing hydration (due to occlusion) does not always increase penetration rates. For example, Bucks et al. (1991) reported that hydration diminished the penetration rate of hydrophilic compounds like hydrocortisone (log octanol/water partition coefficient, or log K_{ow}, of 1.61). In contrast, Wurster & Kramer (1961) observed that occlusive coverings that prevented water loss increased the dermal absorption of some hydrophilic compounds. Increased skin hydration has been cited as the probable cause of the increase in absorption, although in most studies contributions from potentially confounding effects such as increased temperature or accumulation of sweat in the dressing cannot be dismissed (Wurster & Kramer, 1961; Fluhr et al., 1999; Zhai & Maibach, 2001, 2002; Schäfer et al., 2002).

3.5 Reservoir effects

It has long been understood that a substance, instead of passing entirely through the skin, can remain partly in the skin and can act as a reservoir, being released (or not) at a later time (Vickers, 1972; Roberts et al., 2004). This effect has been used in the topical application of medications; for example, salicylic acid was found to be excreted in the urine more slowly when applied topically than when injected intradermally (Guillot, 1954). This is applicable for the more slowly diffusing drugs (i.e. those with long lag times; see chapter 4). The reservoir function of the skin means that the skin can also act as a depot for drugs (or chemicals). The release of the substance can be rapid on appropriate provocation of the skin some time later (e.g. this has been shown with steroids, where an occlusive dressing was applied to the original steroid application site several weeks after the original application) or alternatively using chemical enhancement (Roberts et al., 2004). The duration of the reservoir depends on the nature of the permeant, the vehicle used, the temperature of the skin, and the relative humidity to which the skin is exposed (Vickers, 1972).

Although most studies have emphasized the stratum corneum as a reservoir, viable epidermis, dermis, and underlying tissues may themselves act as reservoirs (Roberts et al., 2004).

Reservoir effects are well documented for several lipophilic compounds (Miselnicky et al., 1988). The water-insoluble fragrance musk xylol showed rapid and significant diffusion from the skin within 72 h after application of a dermal dose (Hood et al., 1996). However, the formation of a skin reservoir for a chemical during percutaneous absorption is not limited to lipophilic chemicals but also applies to polar and non-polar chemicals that bind to the skin during the absorption process (Yourick et al., 2004). Nicotine, caffeine, cationic β-blocking drugs, surfactants, testosterone, malathion, hair dyes, vitamin E, and glycolic and lactic acids have all been reported as forming a skin reservoir (Roberts et al., 2004). Amounts of phenanthrene, benzo[*a*]pyrene, and di(2-ethylhexyl)phthalate remaining in hairless guinea-pig skin after 24 h eventually became available for systemic absorption (Chu et al., 1996). The catechol reservoir formed in skin during a 24-h study with catechol (having good water and lipid solubility) did not decrease (in vivo) or only partially decreased (in vitro) in a 72-h extended study (Jung et al., 2003).

In a set of 19 pesticides tested in the rat in vivo to determine the fate of the skin reservoir, it was found that absorption from the washed skin continued for 15 pesticides at all doses tested.

However, only nine showed an increase in systemic concentrations (Zendzian, 2003).

The potential for a chemical to form a skin reservoir can be at least partially predicted by the extent of protein binding, the rate of penetration through the skin, and the chemical's solubility properties (Miselnicky et al., 1988).

Reservoir characteristics are discussed in section 6.4, and the consequences of reservoir effects for risk assessment are given in section 12.3.

4. SKIN TRANSPORT MECHANISMS AND THEORETICAL CONCEPTS

4.1 Transport through the skin

Percutaneous absorption includes permeation through the epidermis and uptake by the capillary network at the dermal–epidermal junction (see section 2.2). Percutaneous absorption occurs mainly transepidermally (across the stratum corneum intracellularly and intercellularly); for many chemicals, transport through appendages is not usually important in humans (see chapter 3).

Permeation of a chemical through the stratum corneum is basically a diffusion process in which active transport plays no role. The layer with the highest resistance to diffusion is the rate-limiting membrane. For many compounds, the lipophilic stratum corneum is the primary or rate-limiting barrier. However, diffusion through the hydrophilic epidermis and dermis can be rate limiting for very lipophilic materials and/or when the stratum corneum is damaged or affected by disease.

After the chemical diffuses in the mainly aqueous environment (living epidermis and dermis), it is taken up into the cutaneous blood and lymphatic system (resorption). However, if blood flow is insufficient, compounds can accumulate in the viable epidermis, in the dermis, and in deeper tissues.

4.2 Theoretical aspects of diffusion

Diffusion of compounds across a membrane is described by Fick's first law (Crank, 1975):

$$J = -D\frac{\partial C}{\partial x}$$

which states that the flux (rate of transfer per unit area) of a compound (J, mass/cm^2 per second) at a given time and position is proportional to the differential concentration change ∂C over a differential distance ∂x (i.e. the concentration gradient $\partial C/\partial x$). The negative sign indicates that the net flux is in the direction of decreasing thermodynamic activity, which can often be represented by the concentration. Fick's second law describing concentration within a membrane

$$\frac{\partial C}{\partial t} = D\frac{\partial^2 C}{\partial x^2}$$

is derived by combining a differential mass balance in a membrane with Fick's first law and, when considering the skin, assuming that the compound does not bind, the compound is not metabolized, and its diffusion coefficient does not vary with position or composition (Crank, 1975).

Fick's first law can be applied to describe the diffusion processes in the individual layers of the skin, which are treated as pseudo-homogeneous membranes (Scheuplein & Blank, 1971; Dugard, 1977).

For a membrane of thickness h, the flux at steady state (J_{ss}) is given by:

$$J_{ss} = D\,(C_1 - C_2)\,/\,h \qquad \text{[Equation 1]}$$

where C_1 and C_2 are the concentrations of the chemical in the membrane at the two faces (i.e. at $x = 0$ and $x = h$). When used to describe heterogeneous membranes like the stratum corneum, D is an effective diffusion coefficient.

Commonly, the stratum corneum controls dermal absorption, h is the thickness of the stratum corneum, and the concentration at $x = h$ is zero or very small (i.e. $C_2 \approx 0$, which is sometimes called sink conditions). Also, the concentration of chemical at $x = 0$ is in local equilibrium with the vehicle (i.e. $C_1 = K_m \cdot C_v$, in which K_m is the pseudo-homogeneous partition, or distribution, coefficient between the stratum corneum and the vehicle and C_v is the vehicle concentration). Under these conditions, Equation 1 becomes:

$$J_{ss} = D \cdot K_m \cdot C_v\,/\,h \qquad \text{[Equation 2]}$$

The steady-state flux across the skin is sometimes written in terms of the permeability coefficient (K_p) as follows:

$$J_{ss} = K_p \cdot C_v \qquad \text{[Equation 3]}$$

Comparing Equations 2 and 3,

$$K_p = K_m \cdot D / h \qquad \text{[Equation 4]}$$

Note that, although the partition coefficient K_m is unitless, to be consistent with its use in Fick's law, it is the ratio of concentrations in the stratum corneum and vehicle in units of mass/volume (Cleek & Bunge, 1993).

Typically, the steady-state flux J_{ss} and the permeability coefficient K_p are assessed from an in vitro experiment in which the donor concentration of the penetrant is maintained (more or less) constant (i.e. infinite dose conditions), while the receiver phase provides "sink" conditions. Over time, the flux approaches a steady-state value (J_{ss}), and the cumulative amount penetrating the skin increases linearly in time, as illustrated in Figure 5.

The slope of the linear portion of the graph of the cumulative amount penetrated as a function of time represents the steady-state flux J_{ss} (Scheuplein & Blank, 1971; Crank, 1975; Dugard, 1977). As indicated by Equation 3, K_p is the ratio of J_{ss} and the vehicle concentration C_v. The lag time (t_{lag}) is the time intercept of the linear portion of the graph in Figure 5. The time required for the permeation rate across a membrane to reach 95% of the steady-state value is approximately 2.3 times the lag time (96% → 2.4, 97% → 2.5, 98% → 2.8, 99% → 3.2) (Barry, 1983; Bunge et al., 1995). Thus, estimates of steady-state flux and permeability coefficients should include data only from times greater than the time to reach steady state. Including data for times before the steady state is established will lead to a false estimate, usually underestimate, of the permeability coefficient and lag time (Shah, 1993; Schaefer & Redelmeier, 1996; Geinoz et al., 2004). In reality, depletion of the donor phase, the use of non-sink receptor conditions, and a deterioration of the skin over time can occur and result in inaccuracies in steady-state flux and lag time estimations.

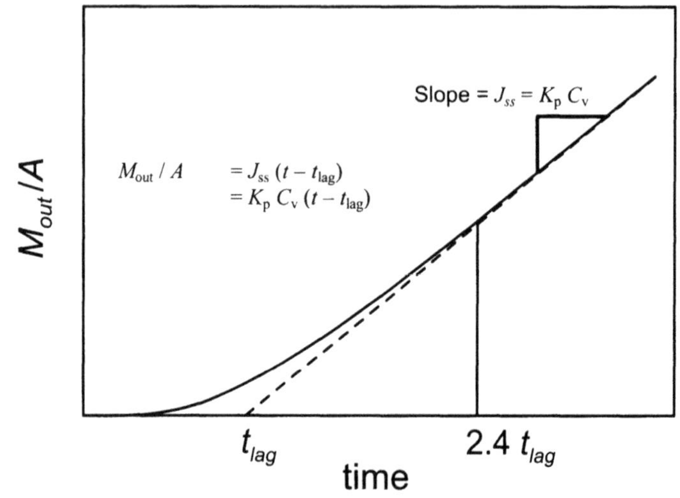

Fig. 5. Illustration of the relationship between the cumulative mass penetrating a membrane area (M_{out}/A) and the steady-state flux, permeability coefficient, and lag time (t_{lag}).

The maximum flux ($J_{max,ss}$) of a solute through a membrane occurs for a pure solid or a saturated solution of a chemical in a vehicle when $C_2 \approx 0$ (Higuchi, 1960; Roberts et al., 2002). At equilibrium, a saturated solution of chemical in a vehicle will be in equilibrium with the saturated concentration of solute in the stratum corneum (S_{sc}). The maximum flux $J_{max,ss}$ is therefore given by Equation 5, which is derived from Equation 1. It is to be noted that $J_{max,ss}$ is also related to the permeability coefficient of a solute in a given vehicle $K_{p,v}$ and the solubility of the solute in that vehicle S_v.

$$J_{max,ss} = S_{sc} \cdot D \,/\, h = K_{p,v} \cdot S_v \qquad \text{[Equation 5]}$$

In principle, higher than maximum fluxes can be observed in intrinsically unstable systems, such as supersaturated solutions.

4.3 Physicochemical factors affecting skin permeation

The physical and chemical properties of a compound and its vehicle have a decisive influence on its permeation through the skin.

4.3.1 Physical state

Thermodynamically, pure powders and saturated liquid solutions of the same compounds have the same driving force for dermal absorption (Higuchi, 1960; Roberts et al., 2002). However, availability to the skin surface may cause the absorption rates to be different. Absorption from dry particulates can occur even without surface moisture (Romonchuk & Bunge, 2003). However, dermal absorption of chemicals in solutions may be more rapid than absorption from particulates. Although data are limited, particle size would be expected to have an effect, with slower absorption rates from larger particles (see also section 12.9 on nanoparticles).

4.3.2 Molecular size/molecular weight

Molecular size is an important factor in membrane permeation (Berner & Cooper, 1984; Cussler, 1997). Theoretically, molecular volume should be a better predictor of flux and the permeability coefficient K_p. However, molecular weight is often used instead, because it is more readily available and unambiguous (i.e. not estimation method dependent) (Patel et al., 2002; Magnusson et al., 2004a). The equations for estimating K_p have been derived from databases containing data on primarily hydrocarbons. For most hydrocarbons, the ratio of molecular weight to molecular volume is nearly constant; thus, K_p estimates based on molecular weight are as good as those based on molecular volume. For dense compounds (e.g. halogenated molecules), molecular weight will be larger relative to molecular volume than for hydrocarbons, and K_p values calculated from equations using molecular weight will be systematically underestimated (Vecchia & Bunge, 2003a). There is good evidence that permeation and maximum flux decrease exponentially with molecular weight (Kasting et al., 1987; Potts & Guy, 1992; Magnusson et al., 2004a). Thus, the extent of absorption of compounds with a molecular weight over 500 daltons through normal human skin is low (Box & Meinardi, 2000).

Using either low-frequency sonophoresis (Tezel et al., 2003) or iontophoresis (Roberts et al., 1998), both of which increase skin permeability, it has been shown for a number of compounds that permeability is also related to solute size and that the optimal pore size utilized by solutes is related to their molecular radii. In low-frequency sonophoresis, larger permeants experience a less tortuous pathway compared with ions and smaller solutes (Tezel et al., 2003).

4.3.3 Maximum flux

The maximum flux of a solute through the skin defines the highest exposure risk for a chemical. Maximum flux, either measured or estimated, is a better guage for dermal absorption than a given physicochemical property of a solute. Hence, neither water solubility nor the octanol/water partition coefficient alone is a reliable indicator of the likelihood of significant dermal absorption. The maximum flux of chemical permeation through skin should occur at the solubility limit of the chemical (Roberts et al., 2002). Thus, one estimate of the maximum flux of a chemical is the product of the chemical's solubility limit in water and the skin permeability coefficient of the chemical from water. Estimated values can also be derived using QSAR equations, as discussed further in chapter 10. For compounds that are completely miscible in water, density of the neat compound can be used in lieu of the water solubility for making preliminary estimates of maximum flux. Generally, dermal absorption would be no larger than the maximum flux, except when the compound or vehicle can damage or alter the skin or in the unusual situation of supersaturated solutions (Davis & Hadgraft, 1991).

For purposes of risk assessment, decisions about whether penetration is important or not must be linked to toxicological potency. For highly potent compounds, the potential for toxic or therapeutic activity might be significant even when maximum flux values are low.

4.3.4 Ionization

Ionized species do not penetrate the skin very well. The stratum corneum permeability coefficients for non-ionized compounds are frequently 1–2 orders of magnitude larger than permeability coefficients for ionized forms of the same compound (Vecchia & Bunge, 2003a). However, ionization effects are less evident in maximum flux estimations (Magnusson et al., 2004a). The exact relationship between the non-ionized and ionized forms would be expected to depend upon the compound and the lipophilicity of the non-ionized chemical, in particular, but also on the vehicle and salt form of the chemical used, as ion pairing may also facilitate ionized drug transport (Hadgraft & Valenta, 2000). Intuitively, the penetration rates for non-ionized and ionized forms of the same chemical should be more similar when the non-ionized species is hydrophilic and less similar when it is lipophilic.

Abraham & Martins (2004) claim that ionization effects are different for acids and bases. They argue that K_p for the neutral form [K_p(N)] of an acid is very much larger than K_p for the ionized form [K_p(I)]. For proton bases, for four different bases studied by two different sets of workers, the $K_p(N)/K_p(I)$ ratios averaged 17.5 (Abraham & Martins, 2004). This conclusion for two of the basic compounds (fentanil and sufentanil) is not accepted by all (e.g. Vecchia & Bunge, 2003a).

4.3.5 *Binding properties*

Permeation through the stratum corneum can be slower than expected for some compounds due to binding. Examples include certain metal ions (particularly Ag^{+}, Cd^{2+}, Be^{2+}, and Hg^{2+}), acrylates, quaternary ammonium ions, heterocyclic ammonium ions, and sulfonium salts. Other potential agents that may have slower than expected permeation possibly due to binding include diethanolamine (Kraeling et al., 2004; Brain et al., 2005), quinines, alkyl sulfides, acid chlorides, halotriazines, and dinitro- or trinitrobenzenes (EC, 2003).

4.4 Concepts of finite and infinite dose

An *infinite dose* is defined as the amount of test preparation applied alone or in a vehicle to the skin such that a maximum rate of absorption of the test substance (per unit area of skin) is achieved and maintained (OECD, 2004a). In principle, the application volume should be large enough that the concentration of the chemical is not depleted. However, an apparent depletion near the skin can occur when the vehicle is sufficiently viscous to cause a diffusional limitation. The infinite dose does not reflect the situation for many occupational exposure scenarios. However, infinite dose exposure can occur in humans. For example, exposure to chemicals such as biocides in swimming pools or bathing water is whole-body infinite exposure. As stated above, the main skin absorption parameters determined in an infinite dose study are the steady-state flux and the permeability coefficient.

Under the conditions of a *finite dose*, the maximum absorption rate may be reached for some of the time, but it is not maintained, or it may not be achieved (OECD, 2004a). The concentration of the chemical in the donor fluid changes due to uptake of the chemical into the skin or evaporation, and it may also change (increase) due to evaporation of the donor fluid. This situation happens in the in vitro cell when it is not occluded, which may be more consistent with most occupational exposures. The finite dose study enables the estimation of both maximal absorption rate (maximal exposure) and total absorption (overall exposure). Simulated examples of the skin permeation rate, cumulative absorption, and vehicle concentration are shown in Figure 6 for infinite, semi-infinite, and finite doses. The semi-infinite dose is simulated as an intermediate case between the true infinite dose (no decrease in concentration in the vehicle during the exposure experiment) and a finite dose (in which the concentration in the vehicle is reduced to less than 10% of the initial concentration after about 20–24 h of exposure).

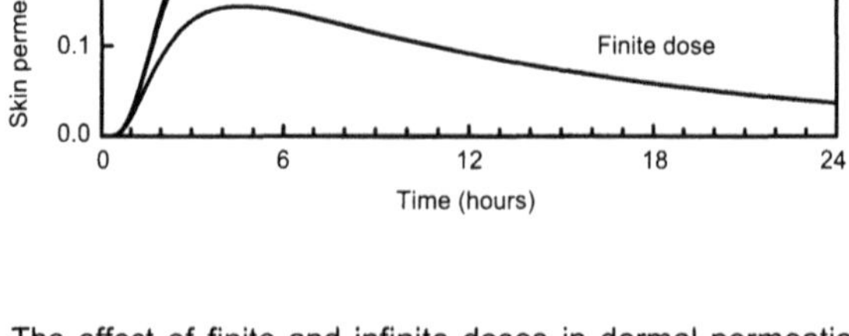

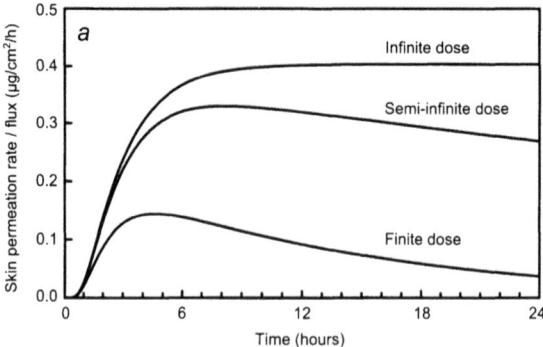

Fig. 6. The effect of finite and infinite doses in dermal permeation. Simulations of a dermal permeation study with a compound having a water solubility of 25 µg/ml and a stratum corneum/water partition coefficient of 200. The compound is dissolved in a water vehicle. a) The skin permeation rate (µg/cm^2 per hour) as a function of time under "infinite" and "finite" dose conditions. (*continued on next page*)

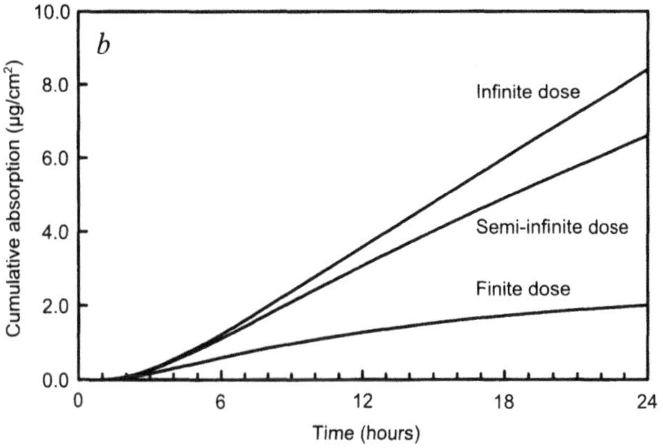

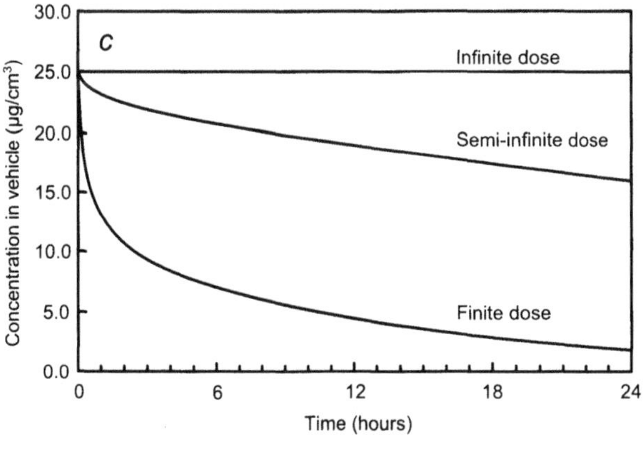

Fig. 6 (*contd*). b) The cumulative amount (µg/cm^2) absorbed through the skin as a function of time under "infinite" and "finite" dose conditions; c) The concentration (µg/cm^3) in the vehicle (donor compartment) as a function of time under "infinite" and "finite" dose conditions (J. Krüse, personal communication, 2005).

5. METABOLISM IN THE SKIN

The skin is a metabolically active organ and contains enzymes that are able to catalyse not only endogenous chemicals such as hormones, steroids, and inflammatory mediators but also xenobiotics, including drugs, pesticides, and industrial and environmental chemicals. Although the metabolism of xenobiotic compounds in the skin is intended to detoxify potentially reactive chemicals by converting lipophilic compounds into polar, water-soluble compounds that are readily excreted into the bile and urine, in some cases a compound may be activated, leading to enhanced local and/or systemic toxicity (Hotchkiss, 1998). Cutaneous activation and detoxification can be a critical determinant of systemic exposure in humans following dermal absorption.

If transport through the viable epidermis is rate limiting *and* the metabolite is less hydrophobic than the parent compound, then percutaneous absorption of the metabolized compound could be faster than (different from) that of the parent compound. Benzo[*a*]pyrene was found to penetrate hairless guinea-pig skin more readily through viable than through non-viable skin, presumably because the more polar metabolites could diffuse more readily through the aqueous viable tissue. Total dermal absorption of benzo[*a*]pyrene through viable skin (67.4% of applied dose) agreed closely with in vivo absorption data (Ng et al., 1992).

It is often assumed that the skin has no first-pass effect, but this is not true for many compounds. Examples include benzo[*a*]pyrene (Ng et al., 1992), nitroglycerine (Wester et al., 1983), herbicide esters (Clark et al., 1993; Hewitt et al., 2000), methyl salicylate (Cross et al., 1997), and parabens (Cross & Roberts, 2000). These effects can not only reduce systemic availability, but also increase localized activity of the metabolites.

Some compounds are designed to be absorbed across the stratum corneum and then metabolized in the skin to the active moiety. Examples of these skin prodrugs and codrugs include retinyl palmitate (Boehnlein et al., 1994), aminolevulinic acid (Donnelly et al., 2005), corticosteroid esters (Hotchkiss, 1998), and the prodrug 5-fluorouracil-triamcinolone-acetonide (Cabral-Lilly & Walters, 2004). Aspects of skin prodrug absorption and metabolism have been reviewed by Hotchkiss (1998) and Benson (2005).

5.1 The drug-metabolizing systems of the skin

The skin contains enzymes that catalyse Phase 1 (e.g. oxidation, reduction, hydrolysis) and Phase 2 (conjugation) reactions (see Table 2). All of the major enzymes important for systemic metabolism in the liver and other tissues have been identified in skin (Pannatier et al., 1978). The specific activities of cutaneous xenobiotic-metabolizing enzymes in the skin, measured in subcellular fractions, are lower than those of their counterparts in the liver (generally 0.1–28% of the activities in the liver for Phase 1; 0.6–50% for Phase 2; see reviews by Kao & Carver, 1990; Hotchkiss, 1998; Hewitt et al., 2000). However, although the basal activities may be relatively low, if the surface area of the skin exposed to the contaminant is very large, the metabolism in the skin is likely to make a contribution to the overall metabolism of the compound following dermal exposure. However, while the skin is a large organ, the only place that metabolism will be important for most substances will be the actual area that is exposed to the chemical.

The extent to which topically applied chemicals will be metabolized depends on the chemical and the enzymes involved. Some chemical groups, such as esters, primary amines, alcohols, and acids, are particularly susceptible to metabolism in the skin (Bronaugh, 2004b).

Esterases are particularly active in the skin, so esters may be extensively, if not completely, hydrolysed to their parent alcohol and acid molecules during skin penetration. Examples of this are the fragrance chemicals such as benzyl acetate as well as the phthalate esters dimethyl-, diethyl-, and dibutylphthalates (Hotchkiss, 1998), retinyl palmitate (Boehnlein et al., 1994), herbicide esters (Clark et al., 1993; Hewitt et al., 2000), and methyl salicylate (Cross et al., 1997). Primary amines are frequently acetylated during percutaneous absorption through the skin (Nathan et al., 1990; Kraeling et al., 1996; Yourick & Bronaugh, 2000). Oxidation/reduction of alcohols and acids and glycine conjugation of acids also commonly occur in the skin (Nathan et al., 1990; Boehnlein et al., 1994). Conjugation with glutathione (Jewell et al., 2000), sulfate (Yourick & Bronaugh, 2000), and glucuronic acid (Moss et al., 2000) also occurs.

Table 2. Some cutaneous metabolizing pathways

Phase 1 reactions	Phase 2 reactions
Oxidation	Glucuronidation
Hydroxylation	Sulfation
Deamination	Glutathione conjugation
Dealkylation	Acetylation
Epoxidation	Amino acid conjugation
Aldehyde oxidation	Methylation
Alcohol oxidation	
Reduction	
Azo reduction	
Nitroxide reduction	
Quinone reduction	
Hydrolysis	
Carboxylester hydrolysis	
Sulfate ester hydrolysis	
Phosphate ester hydrolysis	
Peptide hydrolysis	
Epoxide hydrolation	

[a] From Sartorelli et al. (2000).

Studies in human and rodent skin have shown that cytochrome P450 (CYP1A1/A2) and Phase 2 metabolizing enzymes (e.g. glutathione *S*-transferase) in the skin are localized within specific cell types, particularly in the epidermis and epidermal-derived tissues — namely, sebaceous glands and hair follicles (Pendlington et al., 1994; Hotchkiss, 1998). Lipase, protease, phosphatase, sulfatase, and glycosidase activities have been identified in the stratum corneum; these activities have been linked with the maturation and desquamation processes (Howes et al., 1996). Alcohol dehydrogenase and aldehyde dehydrogenase have also been shown to be present in epidermal basal layers (Haselbeck et al., 1997; Lockley et al., 2004).

5.2 Methodology for evaluating skin metabolism in in vitro systems

The extent of cutaneous metabolism of a chemical applied to the skin is difficult to differentiate in vivo from systemic metabolism, mainly in the liver, using blood and excreta samples. In vitro studies isolate the skin from the metabolic activity in the rest of the body. The use of viable skin is essential. An in vitro flow-through diffusion cell system (Bronaugh & Stewart, 1985; Collier et al., 1989; Bronaugh, 2004a,b; see chapter 6) using a HEPES-buffered Hanks' balanced salt solution as receptor fluid has proved to be an effective method for studying the effect of metabolism of chemicals during percutaneous absorption. Skin metabolism studies have also been conducted in flow-through cells using minimum essential medium to maintain skin viability (Clark et al., 1993) and in an organ culture model (van de Sandt et al., 1993). Additional information can be obtained from studies on the cytosolic fraction of whole and dermatomed skin, such as studies on glycol ethers (Lockley et al., 2004). Skin equivalents have the capacity to metabolize chemicals during dermal absorption, but absorption was also shown to be much faster through skin equivalents than through human skin (Eppler et al., 2005).

Caution should be applied to any in vitro study using skin tissue that claims the tissue is metabolically active. Some enzymes and cofactors, particularly cytochrome P450s and glutathione, deteriorate rapidly ex vivo (in minutes), even in fresh specimens (Jewell et al., 2000). Just because the tissue is used quickly does not "validate" the experiment. Studies would need to show the conversion rate of known standard substrates for the class of enzyme being investigated. Skin penetration is a passive process that can be studied ex vivo. Information on metabolism from the in vitro approach needs to be considered in an in vivo context, and additional in vivo studies may be needed for mechanistic and kinetic understanding.

5.3 Effects of skin metabolism

Cutaneous metabolism may result in:

- activation of inert compounds to toxicologically active species — e.g. polycyclic aromatic hydrocarbons (PAHs), such as benzo[*a*]pyrene (Ng et al., 1992) and 3-methylcholanthrene (Cooper et al., 1980);

- detoxification of toxicologically active chemicals to inactive metabolites — e.g. organophosphorus pesticides, such as diisopropylfluorophosphate, paraoxon (Sartorelli et al., 2000), and propoxur (van de Sandt et al., 1993), and azo dyes (Collier et al., 1993);
- conversion of active chemicals to active metabolites — e.g. drugs such as testosterone and estradiol (Collier et al., 1989); and
- activation of prodrugs (Davaran et al., 2003; Valiveti et al., 2005).

An overview of skin metabolism is given in Hotchkiss (1995, 1998), and metabolism in skin in in vitro absorption studies is described in Bronaugh (2004a). Examples of these studies include azo dyes (Collier et al., 1993), 2-nitro-*p*-phenylenediamine (a dye used in semipermanent and permanent hair dye formulations), where extensive metabolism was found on absorption (Yourick & Bronaugh, 2000), and 2-ethoxyethanol, where no metabolism was observed (Lockley et al., 2002).

5.4 Importance of metabolism for percutaneous absorption

That skin can metabolize compounds before they enter the bloodstream is important for risk assessment purposes and for drug delivery (Howes et al., 1996). However, there are conflicting views concerning the influence of local skin metabolism on percutaneous absorption. Metabolism may not be rate limiting if the compound is stable in the stratum corneum and the stratum corneum limits percutaneous absorption. If the viable tissue is a significant barrier, metabolism of a lipophilic compound in the stratum corneum to a more polar compound might result in enhanced permeation.

Although skin contains enzymes that have the capacity to metabolize glycol ethers localized in the basal layer of the epidermis, the physicochemical properties of the penetrants that result in rapid penetration significantly reduce the potential for first-pass dermal metabolism during percutaneous penetration (Lockley et al., 2004).

However, for compounds that either bind in the skin or, due to their physicochemical properties, stay longer in the skin, the metabolism may be of importance. This may be the case, for example, for PAHs. Seven per cent of the absorbed dose of phenanthrene was biotransformed to the three diol metabolites (*trans*-9,10-dihydrodiol, *trans*-1,2-dihydrodiol, *trans*-3,4-dihydrodiol) in the skin (Ng et al., 1991). These metabolites are not carcinogenic, which correlates with the lack of tumorigenicity of phenanthrene in rodents. In contrast, in skin metabolism studies with benzo[*a*]pyrene, the metabolite identified in the receptor fluid was benzo[*a*]pyrene-7,8,9,10-tetrahydrotetrol, which is the hydrolysis product of the ultimate carcinogen, 7,8-dihydroxy-9,10-epoxy-7,8,9,10-tetrahydrotetrol (Ng et al., 1992). These results agree with the formation of skin tumours following topical administration of benzo[*a*]pyrene. Studies in mouse skin had previously shown that induction of cutaneous drug-metabolizing enzymes can result in a 2- to 3-fold increase in the in vitro permeation of topical benzo[*a*]pyrene (Kao et al., 1985).

The hair dye 2-nitro-*p*-phenylenediamine penetrates both human and rat skin. Under conditions that simulate normal consumer use, approximately 5–10% of the 2-nitro-*p*-phenylenediamine that contacts the skin would be expected to be absorbed. There was extensive metabolism of 2-nitro-*p*-phenylenediamine upon absorption. The extent of metabolism and the metabolic profile depended on species (human, rat) and dosing vehicle (ethanol or hair dye formulation) and also tissue (when compared with results with intestinal tissue) (Yourick & Bronaugh, 2000).

6. IN VITRO TESTS FOR DERMAL ABSORPTION

In vitro methods are designed to measure the penetration of chemicals into and subsequent permeation across the skin into a fluid reservoir and can utilize non-viable skin to measure penetration and permeation only or fresh, metabolically active skin to simultaneously measure permeation and skin metabolism (OECD, 2004a). Permeation across the non-living outer layer of skin, the stratum corneum, is often the rate-limiting step for percutaneous absorption (Dugard & Scott, 1984; Dugard et al., 1984). Permeation of a chemical through the stratum corneum is believed to depend upon permeant-specific factors, such as molecular weight, water and lipid solubility, polarity, and state of ionization (see chapter 4). The permeability properties of the stratum corneum are unchanged after excision from the body, and a good agreement between in vivo and in vitro experiments with the same chemicals has been observed (see chapter 8). Thus, in vitro experiments are appropriate to predict human dermal penetration. Furthermore, such experiments offer a number of advantages over whole-animal or human volunteer experiments, including a saving in time and costs, better reproducibility of results, and less restricted parameter variations (van Ravenzwaay & Leibold, 2004).

In the first part of this chapter (sections 6.1–6.4), various aspects of the methodology of in vitro tests are presented. A discussion of experimental factors that cause variability in results is given in section 6.5.

6.1 Test guidelines

It is only recently that a test guideline for in vitro dermal penetration has been adopted (OECD, 2004a,c). The following descriptions are based on the OECD guideline. A variety of protocols and experimental conditions have been used, and these were later developed into protocols for testing specific substances (e.g. certain regulated chemical substances [USEPA, 2004a]; cosmetics [SCCNFP, 2003b]; see also Appendix 1). The number of different guidelines and protocols have led, in part, to the present problems of comparability of results.

Although OECD (2004a,c) allows the use of various protocols, the guidelines list the issues that investigators must consider in designing their protocols and data analysis, and this should reduce data variation.

6.2 Principles of the standard in vitro tests using skin samples

The test substance, which may be radiolabelled, is applied to the surface of a skin sample separating the two chambers of a diffusion cell (OECD, 2004a). Most common methods for the evaluation of in vitro skin penetration and permeation use diffusion cells, which range in complexity from a simple two-compartment "static" cell (Franz, 1975) to multijacketed flow-through cells (Bronaugh & Stewart, 1985). In all cases, excised skin is mounted as a barrier between the donor compartment and the receptor compartment, and the amount of test chemical and/or its metabolites permeating from the donor to the receptor side is determined as a function of time. The chemical remains on the skin for a specified time under specified conditions, before removal by an appropriate cleansing procedure (OECD, 2004a). Efficient mixing of the receptor phase (and sometimes the donor phase) is essential (Brain et al., 1998a; OECD, 2004a).

6.2.1 Test chambers

Diffusion cells are of the upright/vertical or side-by-side type, with receptor chamber volumes of about 0.5–10 ml and surface areas of exposed membranes of about 0.2–2 cm^2 (Brain et al., 1998a). Both receptor chamber volume and the exposed surface area should be accurately measured and recorded for individual diffusion cells. Vertical cells are useful for studying absorption from semi-solid formulations spread on the membrane surface and are optimal for simulating in vivo performance. The donor compartments can be capped, to provide occlusive conditions, or left open, according to the objectives of the particular study (Brain et al., 1998a). Side-by-side-type (horizontal) diffusion cells are useful for studying mechanisms of diffusion through skin (Bronaugh, 2004b), as the permeation from one stirred solution through the membrane into another stirred solution is measured (Brain et al., 1998a). The chambers in side-by-side diffusion cells are often, but do not need to be, of equal volume. To evaluate topical products intended for human use, standard infinite dose cells in a side-by-side configuration are of limited use; nonetheless, they have been used for this purpose by several authors (Feldmann & Maibach, 1969; Michaels et al., 1975; Bronaugh & Maibach, 1985; Sartorelli et al., 2000; Moss et al., 2002).

Both the vertical and side-by-side cells can be operated in static (i.e. no flow) or flow-through mode.

6.2.1.1 *Static diffusion cells*

The Franz diffusion cell is one of the most widely used systems for in vitro skin permeation studies (Friend, 1992). Franz-type diffusion cell systems are relatively simple in design; the receptor fluid beneath the skin is manually sampled by removing aliquots periodically for analysis (Bronaugh, 2004b). These cell systems may be run as static or as flow-through cells (ECETOC, 1993). With this type of apparatus, any type or any amount of vehicle (within the capacity of the donor chamber) may be applied to the skin. For more realistic exposure scenarios, either 5–10 μl of a liquid vehicle containing the test compound is applied per square centimetre of skin or 2–5 mg of a non-liquid vehicle containing the test compound is applied per square centimetre. An important factor that has to be considered, especially in static diffusion systems, is the solubility of the test compound in the receptor fluid. This may affect the sink capacity and would have an influence on the receptor chamber dimensions or sampling frequency (Brain et al., 1998a). A typical static diffusion cell is shown in Figure 7.

6.2.1.2 *Flow-through cells*

Flow-through cells are characterized by a continuously replaced receptor fluid, which represents, more or less, in vivo conditions. This method can be useful when a permeant has a very low solubility in the receptor medium. Sink conditions are maximized, as the fluid is continually replaced using a suitable pump (at a rate of about 1.5 ml/h) (Brain et al., 1998a). A flow-through diffusion cell system has been developed by Bronaugh & Stewart (1985) (see Figure 8).

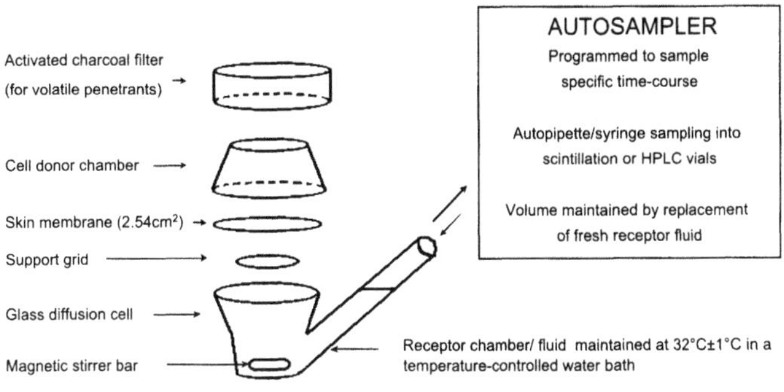

Fig. 7. Design of a typical static diffusion cell for in vitro dermal absorption. HPLC = high-performance liquid chromatography (from OECD, 2004c). [Reprinted with permission]

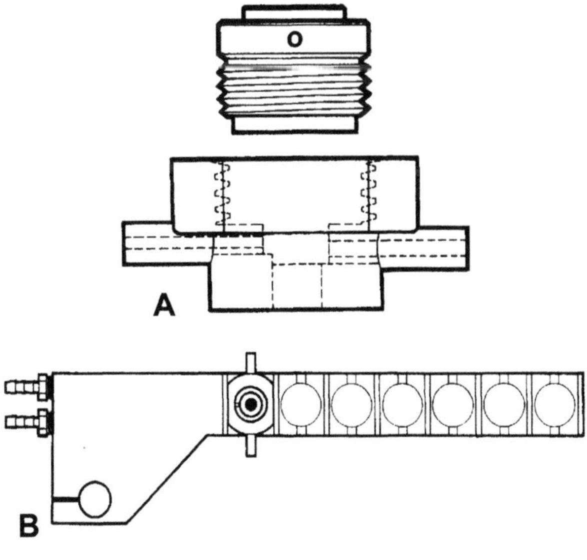

Fig. 8. Flow-through cell and holding block. A — Cross-section of diffusion cell; B — Aluminium holding block used to position cells over vials in a fraction collector and to maintain the cells at a physiological temperature (Bronaugh, 1991). [Copyright (1991) From In Vitro Percutaneous Absorption: Principles, Fundamentals, and Applications by R.L. Bronaugh and H.I. Maibach. Reproduced by permission of Routledge/Taylor & Francis Group, LLC]

The cells were constructed from Teflon and contained a glass window in the receptor chamber for viewing the receptor contents. Several flow-through diffusion cell systems that are comparable to the Bronaugh cell exist (e.g. Clowes et al., 1994; Tanojo et al., 1997).

The receptor fluid and/or the flow rate are selected on the basis of solubility considerations and the volume of the receptor chamber. The criteria that establish a suitable flow rate are 1) that the concentration in the receptor fluid is not greater than about 10% of the solubility limit (as for static diffusion cells) but is large enough to be detected and 2) that there is adequate mixing in the receptor chamber (Skelly et al., 1987). It is important to appreciate that there is a system lag time associated with flow-through cells due to the volume of the receptor chamber and outlet tubing and typically low flow rate used. Either this lag time needs to be corrected for or conditions need to be altered to minimize this effect (Anissimov & Roberts, 2001). One way to minimize the lag effect is by using an adequate flow rate to flush the receptor chamber and outlet tubing completely a number of times each hour (Bronaugh & Stewart, 1985). Automated flow-through systems can allow unattended sampling, and commercial systems are available — for example, the automated in vitro dermal absorption method, which employs tube-shaped skin permeation cells that fit directly into standard 2-ml glass autosampler vials (Moody, 1997, 2000). This procedure permits a quicker sample analysis and minimizes the loss of permeant through evaporation, hydrolysis, and degradation. Good agreement between the automated in vitro dermal absorption method and the Bronaugh procedure was demonstrated using an *N*,*N*-diethyl-*m*-toluamide-based mosquito repellent and permeation through rat skin (Moody, 1997).

6.2.1.3 *Comparison of different in vitro cell systems*

Static cells are simpler in design than flow-through cells, the costs are lower, and they are available in a wide range of surface areas for skin exposure (Bronaugh, 2004b) It also needs to be recognized that adsorption of the test chemical onto the apparatus can occur in the donor and receptor chambers and, where present, the tubing for both types of cell. From a practical point of view, therefore, a further advantage for static cells over flow-through cells is a higher skin:apparatus ratio, which improves the absorption signal and the mass balance distribution assessment. Also, pump problems, connection difficulties, and potential binding of permeant to tubing do not occur using static cells. In contrast to the static cell types, flow-through cells provide the continuous replacement of a nutrient medium necessary to maintain physiological conditions and are therefore recommended for metabolism studies (Bronaugh, 2004a,b).

In several comparative studies, no differences in skin permeability measurements using static and flow-through cells were found (Bronaugh & Maibach, 1985; Bronaugh & Stewart, 1985; Hughes et al., 1993; Clowes et al., 1994). In a multicentre comparison study of in vitro predictions of skin absorption of caffeine, testosterone, and benzoic acid, no differences between static and flow-through diffusion cell systems were observed (van de Sandt, 2004). In another international multicentre study using a standard silicone rubber membrane, there was no consistent pattern of differences between static and flow-through cells (Chilcott et al., 2005).

6.2.2 *Finite/infinite dosing*

There are two dosing regimens: infinite and finite dose (see chapter 4). The finite dose regimen is used where the application is required to be more representative of the "in-use" scenario; the dose solution is applied in a volume sufficient to cover the skin and normally remains unoccluded. Using this regimen, dose depletion is likely to occur. Finite dose experiments may be performed with all types of vertical/upright cells.

In the infinite dose procedure, the dose solution is applied in excess and can be occluded for the duration of the study (Sartorelli et al., 2000; OECD, 2004c). Dose depletion is unlikely to occur.

The dosing regimen and test substance preparation are dictated by the type of experiment being performed. For example, in the assessment of the absorption of a cosmetic ingredient for the purposes of risk assessment, a finite dose with an in-use application protocol and with the test compound in the formulation of interest would be preferred. If a permeability constant is being measured, an infinite dose would be applied for a period sufficient to reach and maintain the steady-state situation.

6.2.3 Skin preparations

6.2.3.1 Choice of skin

The choice of skin depends on the purpose of the test and the availability of skin samples. For risk assessment purposes, human skin is preferred. As stated above, the epidermis is the major barrier for the compound, because once the permeant has transferred across the epidermis, it has access to the cutaneous circulation. In the in vivo situation, the dermis normally has little effect on the dermal absorption of compounds whose rate of absorption is limited by the stratum corneum.

Skin from human and laboratory animal sources can be used. Although the use of human skin samples gives data more appropriate to human in vivo conditions, human skin samples are not always readily available. Further, the use of human skin is subject to national and international ethical considerations (ECETOC, 1993). Typical human in vitro experiments with viable skin involve the use of female abdominal and/or breast skin obtained at autopsy or from cosmetic surgery (Dressler, 1999). Non-viable skin from several anatomical sites of male and female cadavers has also been used.

Rat skin is often used where in vivo toxicological studies have been performed in rats. It is also required for special protocols, such as that for pesticide testing in the USA (USEPA, 1998; Zendzian, 2000). According to the Scientific Committee on Cosmetic Products and Non-Food Products Intended for Consumers (SCCNFP), human skin (abdomen or breast) and pig skin are recommended for cosmetic testing (Steiling et al., 2001; SCCNFP, 2003b). The potential for hydration damage (Bond & Barry, 1988a) and exaggerated effects of enhancers (Bond & Barry, 1988b) with animal skin needs to be recognized. Indeed, Rigg & Barry (1990) concluded: "Wherever possible, human skin should be used in absorption studies and not hairless mouse or snake skin; otherwise, misleading results may be obtained."

Although viable skin (Bronaugh, 2004b) is preferred, especially for metabolism studies, non-viable skin can also be used for certain tests.

OECD Test Guideline 428 (OECD, 2004c) allows a number of skin types and methods of skin preparation for the measurement of dermal absorption in vitro. Indeed, some species are used in in vitro models, either as surrogates for human skin (e.g. pig skin) or to compare absorption between species (e.g. rat and human skin). However, the Task Group's recommendation (see chapter 13) is to use human skin as the gold standard when the dermal absorption potential of a chemical is required for human health risk assessment purposes. Much of the validation type of work in this area has focused on developing in vitro methods to predict dermal absorption in rodents. The emphasis of such work should be to develop consistent and well controlled studies with human skin in order to predict dermal absorption in humans.

6.2.3.2 Preparation of tissue samples

Different methods can be used to prepare skin samples (Brain et al., 1998a; OECD, 2004c):

1) *Full-thickness skin, incorporating the stratum corneum, viable epidermis, and dermis*: Other than for mouse skin, full-thickness skin is normally used for mechanistic studies and should be used in other studies only when justified (OECD, 2004c).

2) *Dermatomed skin, in which the lower dermis has been removed*: Split-thickness skin is produced by dermatoming to obtain skin samples of uniform shape and thickness (Steiling et al., 2001). A dermatome is a surgical instrument that is used to cut skin grafts. Electric and manual dermatomes are generally used. Dermatoming can be carried out from either side of the skin. The trimming and thickness reduction of pig skin are done from the dermis side, in order to generate skin samples with intact stratum corneum and epidermis (Steiling et al., 2001). Skin thickness (usually 0.8–1.0 mm) should be measured by an appropriate method (e.g. using a micrometer gauge; Kenyon et al., 2004a). The skin samples should be prepared and trimmed to fit the diffusion cell (SCCNFP, 2003b).

3) *Epidermal membranes, comprising the viable epidermis and the stratum corneum*: Preparation of an epidermal layer by separation of the epidermis from the dermis using heat is effective for non-hairy skin. (Full-thickness skin is submerged in 60 °C water for approximately 45 s, and the epidermal and dermal layers can be pulled apart with forceps, but the metabolic viability of the skin is destroyed [Bronaugh, 2004b; USEPA, 2004a].) Other methods used to separate the dermis from the epidermis include chemical and enzyme treatment. The use of epidermal membranes may in some cases overestimate human in vivo skin absorption (van de Sandt et al., 2000; SCCNFP, 2003b). According to Bronaugh (2004b), chemical separation techniques and enzyme methods for epidermal separation are limited to use in young rats; according to OECD (2004c), however, they may be used for skin preparation.

4) *Stratum corneum alone*: This tissue is prepared from epidermal membranes by enzyme treatment with trypsin. Stratum corneum membranes are primarily used for mechanistic studies and partition coefficient determination.

The various guidelines indicate that the skin samples that may be used during in vitro studies are split-thickness (200–400/500 μm) (OECD, 2004c; USEPA, 2004a) or, when justified, full-thickness (500–1000 μm) skin preparations (OECD, 2004c). Hairy animal skin should be shaved and the subcutaneous fat removed.

Provided the samples are in their normal state of hydration when cooled, animal and human skin can be stored for up to 1 year at −20 °C (Bronaugh et al., 1986; Steiling et al., 2001). Frozen stored skin may not be suitable for some metabolism studies. Barrier integrity should be evaluated after storage

6.2.3.3 *Checking of barrier integrity*

It has been recommended that before and in some cases after the experiment, the barrier integrity of the skin should be checked by physical methods, such as transepidermal water loss or transcutaneous electrical resistance (Davies et al., 2004; OECD, 2004c; USEPA, 2004a). The barrier integrity of the skin samples may also be checked using the tritium method, where the permeation of tritiated water through the skin is determined and compared with standard values (Ursin et al., 1995; OECD, 2004a,c; USEPA, 2004a). Furthermore, post-study data analysis can be used to identify damaged skin preparations by comparison with the mean absorption data for the other cells (OECD, 2004c).

Typically, skin samples exhibiting a permeability coefficient for tritiated water above 2.5×10^{-3} cm/h are rejected as being out of the "normal" range. In a study to investigate the usefulness of this form of barrier integrity check, K_p values from 1110 human skin samples were found to follow a non-Gaussian distribution (Roper et al., 2004). A rejection criterion of K_p above 2.5×10^{-3} cm/h resulted in rejection of 230 (21%) of these samples. It is likely that many of these rejected samples were atypical rather than "damaged", resulting in an underestimation of absorption in such an individual. There is currently discussion as to whether this rejection criterion is justified (see chapter 12).

6.2.4 Application of test substance

6.2.4.1 Test substance

For practical purposes, the test substance ideally should be radiolabelled (preferably with carbon-14 at a metabolically stable position). However, radiolabelled scintillation counting does not distinguish between metabolites, and further analysis may be necessary. It is essential to determine radiochemical purity (pre- and post-permeation), and the possibility of tritium exchange, where appropriate, should be examined. If radiolabelling is not possible, suitable validated assay procedures must be established for the respective chemicals and metabolites (OECD, 2004c). Current sensitive techniques, such as high-performance liquid chromatography (HPLC), gas chromatography (GC), and liquid chromatography/mass spectrometry (LC-MS), will be useful if a reproducible, validated analytical method to detect the test compounds is available.

Before application of the test substance, various factors that may have an influence on permeation should be considered. These include the nature of the vehicle and the dermal dose (which is dependent on the concentration of the test substance in the vehicle and the applied amount per square centimetre of skin). Other factors include the dosage regimen (finite or infinite) and post-dose conditions, such as occlusion. The test substance application and post-application regimen are dictated by the type of experiment being performed. For example, in the case of the assessment of the permeation of a cosmetic ingredient for risk assessment purposes, a finite dose, with an in-use application time, in the formulation of interest must be used. If a permeability coefficient is being measured, an infinite dose would be applied for sufficient time to reach and maintain steady-state permeation.

6.2.4.2 *Vehicle*

The type of application vehicle will almost certainly have an influence on penetration and permeation (see section 6.5.5). In principle, as shown in Equation 5 (section 4.2), the maximum flux of a solute from saturated solutions across a membrane should be identical and independent of the vehicle, providing the vehicle does not affect the membrane and supersaturation does not occur (Roberts et al., 2002). Hence, in comparing solute fluxes from a given concentration in different vehicles, the vehicle effect may also be seen as a modulation of the vehicle/stratum corneum partition coefficient K_{m}, which is an important factor in determining the rate of penetration of a chemical into the stratum corneum (Scheuplein & Blank, 1971) and may also be the result of a potential direct effect of the vehicle on the stratum corneum. The vehicle/stratum corneum partition coefficient describes the relative affinity of a chemical for the vehicle in which it is applied and the stratum corneum (Suskind, 1977). The more soluble the penetrant in the vehicle, the more likely it is to be retained within the vehicle (Baker, 1986). If the vehicle contains components that directly interact with stratum corneum intercellular lipids, then it is likely that the interaction will cause enhancement or retardation of permeation (Davis et al., 2002). Ideally, the test substance application should be identical to that to which humans or other target species may be exposed. The application may be neat, diluted (ideally with water), or otherwise formulated, as appropriate (OECD, 2004a,c).

6.2.4.3 *Receptor fluid*

The receptor fluid should not act as a rate-limiting step in the permeation process due to limited solubility of the test compound within the medium (i.e. partitioning from the skin to the receptor fluid should be unhindered). In addition, the receptor fluid should not affect skin barrier integrity (OECD, 2004a). For water-soluble compounds, the use of normal saline or an isotonic buffered saline solution is sufficient. For lipophilic test substances, the receptor fluid may contain solvent mixtures such as ethanol:water (although 50% aqueous ethanol may in some cases overestimate permeation), <6% (dependent on permeant) polyoxyethylene[20] oleyl ether in water, or 5% bovine serum albumin (Sartorelli et al., 2000; Bronaugh, 2004b; OECD, 2004a,c). Although 6% polyoxyethylene[20] oleyl ether may have been optimal for the permeants used in the original Bronaugh & Stewart (1984) study, it may not be optimal for all compounds. The surfactant is present to solubilize permeating compounds, and it is possible that lower concentrations may be just as effective at this task for many permeants. When fresh skin is used, the viability of skin can be maintained with either a tissue culture medium or a HEPES-buffered Hanks' balanced salt solution. Care must be taken with surfactants and organic solvents, as the skin barrier can be damaged, particularly when split-thickness skin preparations are used (Bronaugh et al., 1999). It was reported that 1% aqueous solutions of sodium laurate, sodium lauryl sulfate, and other surfactants were found to increase the permeability of water through human epidermis (Sartorelli et al., 2000). However, the enhancement of permeation through addition of permeation-enhancing materials to the receptor phase, although generating incorrect data, will lead to an erroneous but conservative risk assessment.

Ramsey et al. (1994) tested fluazifop-butyl in static diffusion cells with rat and human epidermal membranes using three different receptor fluids: 1) 50% aqueous ethanol, 2) 6% polyoxyethylene[20] oleyl ether in saline, or 3) tissue culture medium. In a comparison with in vivo experiments in rat and human volunteer experiments, use of both 6% polyoxyethylene[20] oleyl ether in saline and tissue culture medium significantly underestimated the in vivo absorption, whereas the use of 50% aqueous ethanol as receptor fluid was adequately predictive of in vivo absorption. Concern has, however, been expressed about ethanol in the receptor phase increasing epidermal permeability (Saunders & Pugh, 2002).

6.2.4.4 *Application dose levels*

For finite dose experiments, an appropriate quantity (1–5 mg/cm^2 or 10 µl/cm^2) of the test preparation should be spread on the skin surface (OECD, 2004c). For infinite dose experiments, typical doses of >10 mg/cm^2 or >100 µl/cm^2 are required to obtain steady-state conditions from which the steady-state flux or absorption rate and the permeability coefficient K_p can be calculated (OECD, 2004c).

6.2.5 *Duration of exposure and sampling time*

The exposure time should reflect in-use conditions. The exposure time may therefore vary between a few minutes for a rinse-off product up to a maximum of 24 h for a leave-on product and 6–8 h for industrial products (OECD, 2004c). For finite dose experiments, the wash-off from the skin should be performed with an aqueous soap solution, and the time of the wash-off determines the exposure (OECD, 2004c). It is important to sample the receptor fluid for at least a 24-h period. Increased exposure times are appropriate only in cases of long lag phases or for infinite applications in order to achieve a steady-state flux (OECD, 2004c). Periods of 24 or 48 h should be adequate to study dermal absorption. Unless adequately preserved, the skin can deteriorate beyond this time. Standard exposure times for test substances in finite dosing experiments are up to 24 h and shorter in the case of rinse-off products (although the measurement of penetration of material continues for at least 24 h).

6.2.6 *Evaluation of the results*

The terminal procedures of an in vitro dermal absorption study are slightly different following infinite and finite dosing experiments. After finite dosing, the mean maximum amount of dermally absorbed material is determined, which requires complete recovery of the test substance (90–110% [OECD, 2004c] or 85–115% [SCCNFP, 2003b]). The quantity washed from the skin, the quantity associated with the skin (and in the different skin layers, if analysed), and the amount present in the receptor fluid should be determined. For infinite dose applications, the steady-state flux is determined and the permeability coefficient K_p calculated; the recovery determination is not relevant to the calculation of K_p, because the only important end-point is the appearance of the test substance in the receptor fluid (OECD, 2004c).

6.2.6.1 Dermal absorption results after finite dosing

The quantity of the test compound and/or its metabolites should be determined in (OECD, 2004a,c):

- applicator (spreader, glass rod, loop, etc.);
- donor chamber (amount removed following rinse procedures);
- dislodgeable dose from the skin surface (terminal washing, sponges, etc.);
- the stratum corneum, when sampled (tape strips, etc.);
- remaining skin sample;
- receptor fluid and receptor chamber; and
- volatile material trap (if present).

For radiolabelled test substances, scintillation counting is performed. For non-radiolabelled substances, HPLC, LC-MS, or GC analysis may be appropriate. According to the OECD, an adequate mean recovery is in the range of 100 ± 10% (100 ± 20% may be acceptable for volatile substances where no trap is present, as lower recovery rates are expected; Bronaugh et al., 1999). Reasons for discrepancies in recovery rates should be explained (OECD, 2004c).

According to OECD Test Guideline 428 (OECD, 2004c), the test substance remaining in the skin should be considered as absorbed unless it can be demonstrated that absorption can be determined from receptor fluid alone. However, when the test substance remains in the skin at the end of the study, it may need to be included in the total amount absorbed (OECD, 2004c).

Cosmetic guidelines suggest that dermal absorption should be expressed as an absolute amount (μg/cm^2 of skin surface) and as a percentage of the amount of test substance contained in the intended dose applied per square centimetre of skin surface (Bronaugh et al., 1999; SCCNFP, 2003b). For cosmetic testing, amounts that are retained by the stratum corneum at the time of sampling are not considered to be dermally absorbed, and thus they do not contribute to the systemic dose (SCCNFP, 2003b). However, for other risk assessments, this amount may be considered as a possible reservoir for systemic dose.

6.2.6.2 *Dermal absorption results after infinite dosing*

The permeability coefficient K_p is calculated (in units of cm/h or cm/s) by dividing the steady-state flux (measured in µg/h per cm^2) by the concentration of the test substance (measured in µg/cm^3) applied to the skin (Bronaugh et al., 1999; USEPA, 2004a).

6.3 Other in vitro methods

6.3.1 *Artificial skin*

Several researchers have developed artificial skin equivalents. Such materials generally attempt to produce membranes that exhibit both hydrophilic and hydrophobic regions and therefore mimic the stratum corneum. Living skin equivalent models have also been employed to assess percutaneous absorption. They consist of skin membranes, including, for example, reconstituted epidermis, grown in tissue culture and used as alternatives to animal tissues (e.g. EpiDerm) (Wagner et al., 2001; Moss et al., 2002). The use of artificial skin is not yet recommended for in vitro testing because of differences in barrier function compared with natural skin (Coquette et al., 2000). Permeation measurements from artificial skin have been inconsistent, making a correlation with either in vitro or in vivo measurements impossible (Heylings et al., 2001; Ponec et al., 2001).

6.3.2 *Tape-stripping technique in vitro*

The methodology of tape stripping is discussed in section 7.2.3. Several studies have evaluated the use of tape stripping in vitro (e.g. for metabolism experiments, see Clark et al., 1993; for dermatopharmacology, see Surber et al., 1999; for establishing a model for in vivo and in vitro experiments, see Trebilcock et al., 1994). In cosmetic testing, it is commonplace to remove the stratum corneum after in vitro testing for mass balance and other purposes.

Table 3 shows the results after in vitro penetration studies with hair dyes, where the amount of test substance identified in the tape-stripped stratum corneum is separated from the amount detected in the deeper skin layers. The test chemicals found in each compartment are shown, and these are related to the amounts recovered as rinses, adsorbed, absorbed, and penetrated (Steiling et al., 2001).

Table 3. Results of percutaneous absorption studies of hair dyes[a]

	% applied dose		
	Hair dye I without developer	Hair dye I with developer	Hair dye II with developer
Rinsings (skin, equipment)	89.5	85.2	88.4
Adsorption (on tape strips)[b]	3.3	2.6	3.7
Absorption (in residual skin)	0.91	0.39	0.63
Penetration (in the receptor)	0.11	0.01	0.30
Bioavailability[c]	1.02	0.40	0.93
Per cent recovery	94.7	89.1	93.0

[a] Adapted from Steiling et al. (2001).

[b] It should be noted that for cosmetic products, the amount remaining in the stratum corneum that can be removed by tape stripping is not considered as systemically available.

[c] Bioavailability: Absorption (in residual skin) + penetration (in the receptor fluid).

6.4 Examination of skin reservoir characteristics

Skin reservoir effects are well documented for steroids (Miselnicky et al., 1988). The reservoir can exist in the stratum corneum, in the viable avascular tissue (viable epidermis), and in the dermis (Roberts et al., 2004) (see also section 12.3).

In order to investigate the potential for the skin to act as a storage depot for a specific substance, a flow-through diffusion cell with either laboratory animal or human full- or split-thickness skin samples may be used. The radiolabelled substance is applied to the skin surface for 5 h. After this time, any remaining test substance is removed by wiping, and the experiment is then left to run for another 15 h, during which time any radioactivity already absorbed into the skin could continue to diffuse across and into the receptor fluid. This receptor fluid is collected every hour (2 ml) for a total of 20 consecutive hours until the end of the experiment. Radioactivity still remaining in the upper stratum corneum may be estimated by tape stripping.

For example, in a study investigating the fate of dihydroxyacetone, 7-(2H-naphtho[1,2-d]triazol-2-yl)-3-phenylcoumarin, and disperse blue 1, the skin penetration and permeation through human and fuzzy rat skin were determined over 24 or 72 h in flow-through diffusion cells (Yourick et al., 2004). Of the three compounds studied, two (dihydroxyacetone and disperse blue 1) formed epidermal reservoirs, and the authors concluded that the amount remaining in the skin should not be considered as absorbed material. On the other hand, the data for 7-(2H-naphtho[1,2-d]triazol-2-yl)-3-phenylcoumarin indicated that this material was spread throughout the epidermis and dermis and, as such, could not be justifiably excluded from the total absorbed dose without further experimentation. These data demonstrate the importance of determining the fate of chemicals remaining in skin.

6.5 Experimental factors affecting dermal absorption in vitro

6.5.1 Species differences

The skins of many species have been evaluated as models for permeation through human skin. Although rat, mouse, and rabbit skins are more permeable than human skin, they have been used to provide a conservative estimate of skin penetration for safety assessments (Feldmann & Maibach, 1969, 1970; Bartek et al., 1972; Scott et al., 1986; ECETOC, 1993; Bronaugh et al., 1999; van Ravenzwaay & Leibold, 2004).

Rat skin was more permeable than human skin to all of a range of tested substances (organic compounds: molecular weight = 231–466 g/mol; aqueous solubility = 0.057–600 000 mg/l; log K_{ow} = 0.7–4.5), with a mean difference of 10.9-fold (van Ravenzwaay & Leibold, 2004). Lipophilic compounds showed the highest penetration rates through rat skin in vitro (van Ravenzwaay & Leibold, 2004). However, the mean value of 10.9-fold should be treated with caution because of the differences in the experimental protocols between in vitro human and in vivo rat evaluations.

Table 4 shows the in vitro absorption of tritiated water (a small polar molecule) and ^{14}C-labelled paraquat dichloride (a fully ionized divalent cation) through human and various laboratory animal skin samples (Scott et al., 1986). In another study, rat skin was shown to be 2.9- to 6.3-fold more permeable than human skin in vitro to trimethylamine (log K_{ow} = 0.16; aqueous solubility = 8.9×10^5 mg/l) (Kenyon et al., 2004a).

Table 4. In vitro absorption of tritiated water and ^{14}C-labelled paraquat dichloride through human and animal skin[a]

Species	Strain	Permeability coefficient (K_p) (cm/h × 10^5)	
		Water	Paraquat
Human		93	0.7
Rat	Wistar Alpk/AP	103	27
	Hairless rat	103	36
	Nude rat	152	35
Mouse	Alpk/AP	144	97
	Hairless mouse	350	1066
Rabbit	New Zealand White	253	80
Guinea-pig	Dunkin-Hartley	442	196

[a] Adapted from Scott et al. (1986).

In their review of rat permeability coefficients for compounds from water, Vecchia & Bunge (2005) found the average ratio of the permeability coefficient for rat skin to the permeability coefficient for human skin to be about 2. This study also examined hairless mouse, hairless rat, and snake skin permeability coefficient data. They reported that, on average, hairless mouse skin is 3.1 times more permeable than human skin, apparently independent of K_{ow}, but perhaps weakly dependent on molecular size.

6.5.2 Temperature

When carrying out in vitro experiments, the skin must be maintained at the physiological temperature of 32 ± 1 °C (OECD, 2004a,c; USEPA, 2004a). Since diffusion is a temperature-dependent process, alteration in skin temperature will affect the absorption process (OECD, 2004a). In the in vitro human skin database evaluated by Vecchia & Bunge (2003a), a statistically discernible difference between the permeability coefficients measured at different temperatures was observed. It has also been observed that, for the same heating bath temperature (in this case, it was 35 °C), the average temperature of the diffusion cells (average of receptor and donor solutions) was different for the configurations of the flow-through and static cells examined, which led to a measurable difference in the permeability across a silicone rubber membrane (Romonchuk & Bunge, 2004). The authors recommended that such experiments be conducted isothermally.

6.5.3 *Occlusion*

The normal exposure situation is most accurately simulated by open unoccluded conditions, because in most instances human skin may be protected but not occluded during exposure. In certain cases, occlusion will be more representative of occupational exposure (e.g. protective gloves, etc.). Unoccluded conditions can avoid the skin barrier modulation caused by excessive hydration, which, in most cases, increases the penetration rate (Kligman, 1983; Bronaugh & Stewart, 1985; Baker, 1986; ECETOC, 1993). A 5- to 10-fold increase in permeability of the stratum corneum was noted when the skin was occluded (Sartorelli et al., 2000). However, volatile substances may evaporate during unoccluded testing, and, because of the dosage regimen, infinite dosing experiments can be done only under occluded conditions (Bronaugh, 2004b; OECD, 2004c). In a dermal absorption study with catechol applied in ethanol, occlusion resulted in 78% of the applied dose permeating into the receptor fluid, compared with 55% in dermal samples that were not occluded (Jung et al., 2003).

6.5.4 *Thickness of skin*

The thickness of the skin sample used in in vitro studies may have an influence on the permeation of the test chemical. Cnubben et al. (2002) found that permeation through viable full-thickness skin membranes was much less than permeation through only the epidermis. In this investigation, the authors studied the in vitro skin penetration of [^{14}C]*ortho*-phenylphenol (log K_{ow} = 3.28) through human and rat viable skin, human and rat epidermal membranes, and perfused pig ears (four to six skin membranes were used per experimental group). Human skin was obtained directly after abdominal surgery, and rat skin was obtained from male albino Wistar Outbred rats. Rat (from Sprague-Dawley rats with clipped dorsal and flank skin) and human epidermal membranes were prepared by overnight immersion of the skin in a solution of 2 mol of sodium bromide per litre containing 0.01% sodium azide. Human and rat epidermis showed a marked higher cumulative permeation (μg/cm^2) than human and rat full-thickness viable skin (Figure 9).

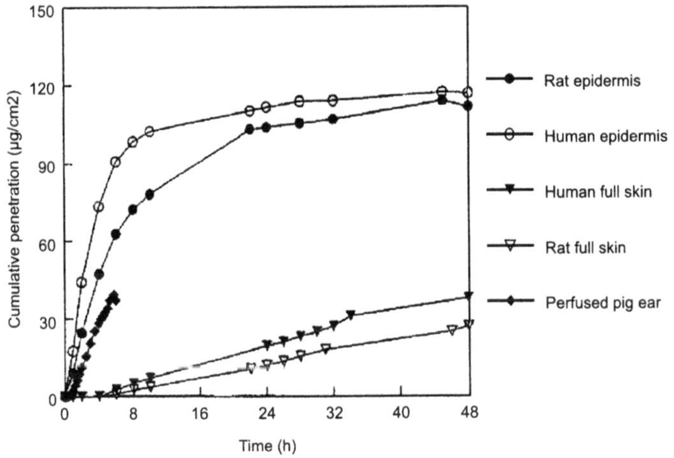

Fig. 9. In vitro skin penetration expressed as cumulative amount reaching the receptor fluid (from Cnubben et al., 2002). [Reprinted from Regulatory Toxicology and Pharmacology, Vol. 35, No. 1, N.H. Cnubben et al., Comparative in vitro–in vivo percutaneous penetration of the fungicide *ortho*-phenylphenol, Pages 198–208, Copyright (2002), with permission from Elsevier]

The influence of skin thickness (0.5–1.3 mm) on percutaneous penetration has been studied using caffeine, testosterone, butoxyethanol, and propoxur by Wilkinson et al. (2004) (EDETOX, 2004). Some differences in the maximum flux and the cumulative doses in receptor fluid, dependent on skin thickness, were seen. This was because the relationship between skin thickness and permeant physicochemical properties is complex (Wilkinson et al., 2004, 2006). Vecchia & Bunge (2003a) also examined whether there were any statistically significant detectable differences between experiments that used different skin layers. Their conclusion was consistent with the observations of Wilkinson et al. (2004, 2006).

6.5.5 *Further observations on application vehicle effects*

Because the solubility of a permeating chemical is usually different in different vehicles, the flux of a compound presented to the skin at the same concentration in different vehicles should be different. If the compound is instead presented to the skin at the same saturation ratio, the flux will be the same, provided the vehicle itself does not alter the skin barrier significantly. As a result, the permeability coefficient K_p, which is the ratio of the flux to the concentration, can be quite different for different vehicles, even if the vehicle does not change the skin, simply because the solubility is different. So, it is not surprising that testosterone was found to have a higher K_p when applied in water, in which it has low solubility, than when applied in petrolatum jelly or ethylene glycol, in which it has higher solubility (Bronaugh & Franz, 1986). The in vitro skin permeability values of caffeine were similar for petrolatum jelly and the water vehicle, but lower for ethylene glycol.

In a recent investigation with a flow-through system, the permeability of [^{3}H]ricinoleic acid — a machine cutting fluid ingredient — through silastic membranes and porcine skin was significantly reduced when it was applied in polyethylene glycol ethers with several additives (2% triazine, 5% triethanolamine, 5% linear alkylbenzene sulfate) compared with several mineral oil mixtures. This is surprising, as these additives are dermal irritants and should theoretically enhance solute permeability. The fact that the opposite was observed suggests that the mixture interaction is more physicochemical in nature and probably not related to the chemical-induced changes in the biological membrane when skin was exposed to these cutting fluid mixtures (Baynes & Riviere, 2004).

The cumulative percutaneous penetration of a ^{14}C-labelled sunscreen, octyl salicylate, in two different formulations (hydroalcoholic lotion and oil/water emulsion), determined using human epidermal membranes prepared from skin obtained from autopsy, was very similar in each case (1.58 µg/cm^2 over 48 h). However, the amount of applied material remaining in the epidermal membranes at 48 h was markedly higher for the hydroalcoholic solution (32.77%) than for the oil/water emulsion (17.18%) (Walters et al., 1999).

Use of isopropyl myristate may be necessary for lipophilic compounds (USEPA, 2004a), but difficulty in extrapolation to test results from exposure conditions involving other vehicles should be acknowledged. USEPA (1992) discussed theoretical relationships that could be used to translate permeability coefficients measured from one vehicle to another vehicle. The approach is to multiply the measured K_p by the ratio of the solubility of the chemical in the vehicle of concern to the solubility of the chemical in the test vehicle.

7. IN VIVO TESTS FOR DERMAL ABSORPTION

This chapter is an overview of the methodology for in vivo tests for dermal absorption. Although some examples are given, this is only a small part of the literature available on this subject. For a compilation of available studies, the reader is referred to databases such as that of EDETOX (undated).

The in vivo methods allow the determination of the extent of cutaneous uptake as well as systemic absorption of the test substance. The main advantage in performing an in vivo study rather than an in vitro study is that the in vivo study uses a physiologically and metabolically intact system (OECD, 2004a,b). In vivo dermal penetration studies are carried out in laboratory animals, usually rodents, and in human volunteers. The latter has been widely used for human pharmaceuticals and, to a more limited extent, for other chemicals. In vivo studies in humans are the gold standard. The conduct of any in vivo study has ethical issues. The main disadvantage of using laboratory animals is that they have different skin permeability and systemic disposition compared with humans. Further, in animals, the dosing site must be protected from grooming behaviour (leading to the disappearance of topical applied compound and, in some cases, oral intake of the test compound) or from contact with the cage. Care needs to be taken to avoid discomfort of the animals.

7.1 Laboratory animal studies

The rat is the most commonly used species for animal in vivo studies, having the advantage that information from other toxicity and toxicokinetic studies is mostly obtained from this species. The male rat is the species and sex required for dermal absorption studies according to the USEPA (1998); however, OECD (2004b) states that other animal species can be used when they have been shown to have skin absorption more similar to that of humans than the rat. It is known that data from rat studies generally overestimate human skin absorption (ECETOC, 1993). Monkeys and pigs show dermal absorption similar to that of humans, but the disadvantages of employing these two animal models are the relatively high maintenance costs and the possible handling difficulties. Other animal models include hairless rats (Simonsen et al., 2002) and mice and fuzzy rats (Klain & Reifenrath, 1991).

There are three classes of in vivo animal studies: 1) in which a compound is measured in blood or excreta, 2) in which material is measured in the skin by biopsy or some other method, and 3) in which the compound is measured in all tissues (residue analysis). Determination of dermal absorption should be based on mass balance considerations.

7.1.1 Test guidelines for laboratory animal studies

It is only recently that the OECD adopted the guideline for in vivo dermal absorption (OECD, 2004a,b). This is similar to the guideline published by the USEPA (1998) for pesticides; however, the standard OECD protocol requires considerably fewer animals, since the number of exposure intervals and the number of dose levels are lower than in the USEPA (1998) protocol. Both protocols are being used for testing industrial chemicals and pesticides. Zendzian (2000) reported that over 160 pesticides have been evaluated on the basis of the USEPA (1998) protocol.

7.1.2 Principles of the standard in vivo tests

The test chemical is applied to a designated area of skin in an appropriate format (e.g. in solvent or formulation for a defined period). Body fluids, tissue, or excreta are collected at predefined intervals, and the quantity of chemical and/or metabolite in the samples is measured by a suitable analytical procedure (Wester & Maibach, 1999b). The collection of expired air should be considerd when there is information that the chemical and/or its metabolite are excreted by this route. The analytical method of choice must be appropriately sensitive, since percutaneous absorption is often low (ECETOC, 1993). In vivo tests are sometimes required for regulatory purposes for registration of pharmaceuticals and pesticides (e.g. USEPA, 1998).

7.1.2.1 *Preparation of the application site*

At least 24 h before treatment, the application site should be prepared (OECD, 2004b). (USEPA [1998] specifies 24 h for measuring dermal absorption from pesticides.) In the rat, for example, the hair on the shoulders and the back is removed with animal hair clippers; shaving of the application site should be avoided, in order to avoid abrasions, which will artificially increase dermal penetration (OECD, 2004a,b). If the skin is washed prior to application (with water or a mild detergent), the possibility of skin or barrier property modifications has to be carefully considered (OECD, 2004c).

7.1.2.2 *Dose levels*

Skin absorption of chemicals applied in a finite dose formulation is generally not linearly related to dose, the flux being lower at the higher dose per unit area. It is therefore important that the selected doses span the range of doses expected in field exposure. These should be determined on the basis of quantity per unit area of exposed skin (mg/cm^2). The USEPA (1998) recommended that four, but at least three, doses should be used, which should be at log intervals. OECD Test Guideline 427 (OECD, 2004b) mentions that the test substance preparation should be the same (or a realistic surrogate) as that to which humans may be exposed. For pesticides, most often the concentrate formulation and one or two application dilutions are tested.

7.1.2.3 *Application of the test substance to the skin*

The test substance preparation, which ideally is radiolabelled in a metabolically stable position, is applied to 5–10% of the surface of the skin (for rats with body weight 200–250 g: 10 cm^2) (USEPA, 1998). The OECD (2004b) guidance specifies application of 10 $\mu l/cm^2$ for a liquid substance and 1–5 mg/cm^2 for a solid. This specification of the volume is based on an unconstrained application (i.e. to prevent the solution from running over a larger area) if one were trying to simulate a skin splash. Other volumes per area might be used if the area is constrained by a ring or other means that prevents any spreading of the chemical outside the defined area and prevents the animal from interfering with the application site. A common procedure uses a ring of an inert material (rubber, polytetrafluoroethylene), which is glued to the skin over the clipped area, before application of the test formulation, using cyanoacrylate adhesive to confine the treated area (OECD, 2004b). The application system must be covered with, for example, a nylon gauze, which may be glued over the ring to protect the test preparation against unintentional removal or spreading. Some laboratories use a collar or rubber tubing placed behind the forelegs or neck of the animals. The use of a jacket with a plastic shield to cover the site is also acceptable. As long as one can prevent the animal from grooming the treatment site and prevent excessive loss of material from the site into the cage, there is no restriction (within ethical limits) as to what can be used.

7.1.2.4 *Duration of exposure*

In general, the extent of absorption is directly related to the duration of application (Roberts & Walters, 1998). The duration of exposure is the time between application and removal of the skin by skin washing. OECD Test Guideline 427 (OECD, 2004b) requires an exposure period relevant to the occupational situation (typically 6 or 24 h). The USEPA (1998) guideline requires evaluation with time (in the standard protocol: 0.5, 1, 2, 4, 10, and 24 h). The animal should be observed for clinical signs of toxicity throughout the duration of the study, and the treated skin should be observed for visible signs of irritation (OECD, 2004b).

After the exposure period, the test preparation is removed by an appropriate cleansing procedure. In the USEPA (1998) protocol, the animals are sacrificed at this time point. In the OECD (2004b) protocol, the animals are housed individually in metabolism cages after the skin is washed. Excreta and (if appropriate) exhaled air are collected until sacrifice of the animals.

7.1.2.5 *Sacrifice and time of termination*

OECD Test Guideline 427 (OECD, 2004b) mentions that animals will be sacrificed at different time intervals — for example, at the end of the exposure period (typically 6 or 24 h) and at subsequent occasions (e.g. 48 and 72 h). The USEPA (1998) protocol requires that the animals be sacrificed at the exposure intervals, which, in the standard study, are 0.5, 1, 2, 4, 10, and 24 h. In both guidelines, blood and various other samples are collected for analysis.

7.1.2.6 *Evaluation of the results*

The quantity of non-pharmaceutical chemical or its metabolites must be determined in (OECD, 2004c):

- dislodgeable dose from the skin surface (washing water);
- skin from the treated and non-exposed site (stratum corneum, epidermis, and dermis);
- dislodgeable dose and desquamated skin (from protective dressing post-exposure);
- urine, faeces, and cage washing;
- expired air, if applicable (>5% volatile metabolites of applied dose);
- blood and remaining carcass; and
- solvent washing of contaminated material and application system.

An adequate mean recovery is in the range of 100 ± 10%, although this recovery is higher than is often observed. Recoveries outside the given range should be justified.

The dermal absorption is usually given as a percentage of the dose applied and is obtained by addition of amounts recovered from urine, faeces, and cage washing, expired gas, blood and remaining carcass, and dose skin. Tape stripping can be performed in order to obtain information on the test chemical deposition (Trebilcock et al., 1994).

If the animals are not sacrificed, then an indirect measure of absorption (by monitoring urine, faeces, or blood) is required, including some sort of adjustment to account for material that is absorbed but not measured in the fluid that is monitored. Where possible, pharmacokinetic analyses are undertaken to estimate the rate and the extent of absorption. The overall extent of absorption can be defined in terms of the absolute bioavailability — i.e. the fraction F of the dose reaching the systemic circulation intact after extravascular administration. This bioavailability is best determined by comparison with plasma/blood or urine levels of unchanged solute achieved with the intravenous administration of the solute. Normally, either the area under the plasma concentration–time profile (AUC) or the amount excreted unchanged in the urine (A_u) from the time of administration to infinite time is used to define F (Roberts & Walters, 1998):

$$F = [A_{u,topical}/dose_{topical}] / [A_{u,iv}/dose_{iv}]$$

$$= [AUC_{topical}/dose_{topical}] / [AUC_{iv}/dose_{iv}]$$

The percentage of dermal absorption can therefore be calculated from:

Percentage dermally absorbed =

$$\frac{\text{total \% excreted after topical dose}}{\text{total \% excreted after intravenous dose}} \times 100$$

In the absence of intravenous studies, the percentage absorbed has to be estimated by mass balance, which is given by the amount excreted divided by the amount applied (Roberts & Walters, 1998).

7.2 Studies with human volunteers

Studies with human volunteers provide definitive data for the assessment of the absorption of chemicals through human skin; for technical and ethical reasons, however, their use is limited and their conduct is closely regulated (Declaration of Helsinki, 1964 and updates: World Medical Association, 2004; and the International Conference on Harmonization Guideline for Good Clinical Practice: ICH, 1996). The use of radiolabelled compounds for human studies is subject to further regulation by the International Commission on Radiological Protection (http://www.icrp.org). Dermal absorption in vivo can be assessed using different approaches, such as plasma and excreta assessments, breath analysis, tape stripping of the stratum corneum, microdialysis, and radiography. Each of these approaches encounters specific problems, which will be discussed in more detail in the following sections.

7.2.1 Assessment using plasma, excreta, and breath analysis

7.2.1.1 *Methodology*

In vivo experiments are often used as a gold standard for alternative methods, such as in vitro studies and predictive modelling. It is therefore important that for the purpose of comparison, in vivo experiments deliver the same parameters — e.g. absorption rate, permeability coefficient K_p, etc. Deconvolution of pharmacokinetic data can be used to estimate the absorption rate profiles of topically applied chemicals using plasma data and comparison with intravenous plasma data. Several methods of performing pharmacokinetic deconvolution are available (e.g. Yu et al., 1996; Levitt, 2003). The extent of absorption can be defined by the equations given in section 7.1.2.6. However, in most in vivo studies for chemicals, the intravenous data are not usually available, and a preferred approach is the use of mass balance or data from another administration route. In the case of mass balance, where the amount recovered (in the stratum corneum and in urine) is compared with the amount applied, only the average absorption rate can be estimated (Roberts & Walters, 1998). By use of another route of administration, the relative extent of absorption can be compared (Mráz & Nohová, 1992; Brooke et al., 1998), or the average absorption rate can be estimated if the amount administered by the other route is known. However, a preferable method would be to estimate dermal absorption rate profiles in a similar manner as described for intravenous dosing — e.g. by using inhalation with a known input rate. This method has been widely used for the determination of dermal absorption of liquids (Kezic et al., 2001; Jakasa et al., 2004b), solids (including those dissolved in an appropriate vehicle), and vapours (Kezic et al., 2000, 2004).

The chemical is usually applied on the forearm or back skin. For vapours, however, whole-body exposure has also been used. Pharmaceutical preparations would be applied on the site of intended use.

7.2.1.2 *Examples of in vivo human volunteer studies*

Some examples of compounds applied in liquids include hormones (e.g. Feldmann & Maibach, 1969), drugs (e.g. Dehghanyar et al., 2004; Martin et al., 2004), hair dyes (e.g. Wolfram & Maibach,

1985; Dressler, 1999), disinfectants (e.g. Turner et al., 2004), fragrances (e.g. Ford et al., 2001; Hawkins et al., 2002), industrial chemicals (e.g. Hanke et al., 1961, 2000; Dutkiewicz & Tyras, 1967, 1968; Feldmann & Maibach, 1970; Dutkiewicz et al., 2000; Kalnas & Teitelbaum, 2000; Kezic et al., 2000), and pesticides and herbicides (e.g. Feldmann & Maibach, 1974; Dick et al., 1997a,b; Garfitt et al., 2002a,b,c; Meuling et al., 2005; Ross et al., 2005).

In contrast to liquids, there are fewer studies on dermal absorption of vapours in humans. A number of early studies were conducted in the former Soviet Bloc and nearby countries, including studies on benzene (Hanke et al., 1961, 2000), aniline (Dutkiewicz & Piotrowski, 1961), phenol (Piotrowski, 1971), *m*-xylene, styrene, toluene, 1,1,1-trichloroethane, and tetrachloroethene (Riihimaki & Pfaffli, 1978). More recent compounds studied include xylene, toluene, 2-butoxyethanol, tetrahydrofuran, methyl ethyl ketone, 1-methoxypropan-2-ol, *N,N*-dimethylformamide, and *N,N*-dimethylacetamide (Johanson & Boman, 1991; Mráz & Nohová, 1992; Kezic et al., 1997, 2004; Brooke et al., 1998; Nomiyama et al., 2000, 2001).

The results of these studies have shown that for some substances, such as the glycol ethers, skin uptake from vapours may be an important contributor to the total uptake; for example, a 5–10% contribution to the total body burden was seen for 1-methoxypropan-2-ol (Brooke et al., 1998). Also, other studies demonstrate good dermal absorption of various glycol ether vapours (Johanson & Boman, 1991; Kezic et al., 1997; Jones et al., 2003; Jakasa et al., 2004b) or, to a lesser extent, of xylene (Kezic et al., 2004). About 40% contribution to the total body burden was reported for *N,N*-dimethylformamide and *N,N*-dimethylacetamide (Mráz & Nohová, 1992; Nomiyama et al., 2000, 2001).

7.2.1.3 *Biomonitoring of occupational exposure*

Biomonitoring gives an indication of the internal dose of a chemical by monitoring levels of chemicals and metabolites in the blood, urine, or breath. For practical and ethical reasons, usually urine samples are monitored (IPCS, 2001). However, the amount of exposure by the dermal route may not be distinguishable from that by the inhalation or ingestion route. Human volunteer data in which exposure is controlled will allow establishment of the relationship between levels in the biological fluids and the dermally applied dose (e.g. Jakasa et al., 2004b).

Unless a worker is breathing clean air, it may not be possible to separate dermal exposure from inhalation exposure. Observation of the worker and work practices is important for defining the routes of exposure.

Biological monitoring of urinary metabolites generally reflects metabolism in the liver rather than skin metabolism, even for a dermally absorbed dose. Dermal metabolism could potentially be distinguished if the dermal metabolic profile differs from the liver metabolic profile, as suggested for cypermethrin by Woollen et al. (1992), or, if dermal absorption is extensive, by comparison with the urinary excretion of an intravenous dose. Generally, only one urine sample is available for analysis, taken at the end of shift or later for chemicals with a long half-life. Theoretically, the urinary profile of a chemical absorbed through the skin would be more delayed than the urinary profile of the chemical taken up by inhalation due to the lag time in dermal absorption; thus, if two or more samples are available and an excretion profile were obtained, it might be possible to deduce whether most of the exposure was by the dermal route. However, this approach has not been fully investigated.

Interindividual variability in liver metabolism, which may be up to 10-fold, may contribute to variability in urinary parent and metabolite levels. Knowledge of the chemical half-life, metabolism profile, clearance, and the enzymes involved is required to interpret biological monitoring data.

7.2.2 *Cutaneous microdialysis*

Cutaneous microdialysis is an in vivo sampling technique used for the measurement of endogenous and exogenous substances in the extracellular space beneath the skin using perfused dialysis. This technique has been used in human volunteers (Anderson et al., 1998; Benfeldt, 1999; Schnetz & Fartasch, 2001; Korinth et al., 2004; Joukhadar & Muller, 2005) and in laboratory animal experiments (Benfeldt, 1999; El Marbouh et al., 2000; Mathy et al., 2004). The microdialysis system consists of microinjection pumps and microdialysis probes with polyurethane (semipermeable) membranes (El Marbouh et al., 2000), which may be implanted into blood vessels, the dermis, or the subcutaneous tissue. The blood flow in a vessel underneath the skin surface is mimicked by continuously passing a receptor fluid through the microdialysis tubing and collecting it in a collector. Two methods are commonly used: 1) one requiring two puncture sites and referred to as a push-through method (Figure 10), and 2) a single-puncture system with inlet and outlet of the same site. Using these methods, it is possible to measure the local concentrations of a test compound in the dermis and to monitor percutaneous absorption of various substances (El Marbouh et al., 2000).

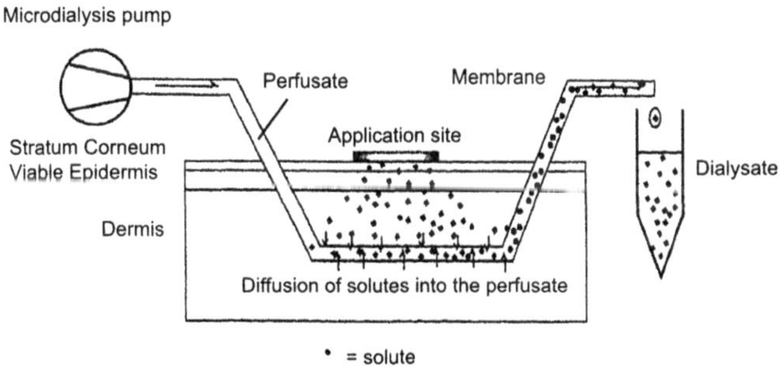

Fig. 10. Scheme of the microdialysis system (from Schnetz & Fartasch, 2001). [Reprinted from European Journal of Pharmaceutical Sciences, Vol. 12, No. 3, E. Schnetz & M. Fartasch, Microdialysis for the evaluation of penetration through the human skin barrier — a promising tool for future research?, Pages 165–174, Copyright (1991), with permission from Elsevier]

Dermal absorption kinetics and dermal metabolism may be studied using this technique. The results are usually expressed in terms of relative recovery (Leveque et al., 2004), as the quantity of a compound recovered across the microdialysis tubing is only a fraction of the quantity present in the tissue.

Microdialysis has been used to investigate the influence of penetration enhancers, vehicles, or iontophoresis on percutaneous absorption in vivo in rats. The experiments in volunteers are limited to 6–8 h, and most studied compounds are fast penetrating. One problem with microdialysis is the calibration of the technique (e.g. the assessment of the recovery). This can be determined using a parallel in vitro approach. The position of the tubing should be determined for standardization using ultrasound (Muller et al., 1997; Anderson et al., 1998) or related techniques. Microdialysis normally uses an aqueous perfusate and is used to estimate water-soluble substances. Dialysates containing albumin have been used in estimating the dermal absorption of other more lipophilic solutes. A second problem is the variability associated with dermal microdialysis (McCleverty et al., 2006). Care must be taken with study design, using, where possible, each subject as his or her own control twice to remove subject-to-subject variability in sample size estimations and to provide an estimate of the intrasubject variability.

7.2.3 *Tape stripping*

Tape stripping of human stratum corneum has frequently been used for investigation of skin penetration, barrier function, and the factors involved in skin pathologies (Bashir et al., 2001; Choi et al., 2004; Loffler et al., 2004). The method is simple, inexpensive, and minimally invasive and can be used in both humans and laboratory animals.

In a tape-stripping experiment, a predetermined area of skin is exposed to a chemical for a fixed application period. After exposure, stratum corneum from the exposed skin site is removed sequentially by successive application of adhesive tape. The amount of the substance recovered by the tape is then analysed using an appropriate analytical method. A comparison of various tape-stripping methods is given in Choi et al. (2004), which shows the variance in the methods used. The number of tape strips needed to remove a given fraction of the stratum corneum varies with the type of tape (Bashir et al., 2001), experimental factors such as the pressure applied during application, peeling force for removal, and anatomical site, as well as age, sex, and possibly ethnicity of the subject (Palenske & Morhenn, 1999; Loffler et al., 2004). It has also been shown that the adhesive properties of the tape as well as the cohesion of the corneocytes may be influenced by the vehicle (Surber et al., 1999), and this will also affect the number of strips required to completely remove the stratum corneum.

Despite these complications, some protocols have specified the number of tape strips that should be collected. Rougier et al. (1999) recommended that the capacity of the stratum corneum reservoir for each compound be defined as the sum of the amounts found in the first six strippings. The USFDA (1998) guidance specifies that 12 tape strips should be collected, and OECD (2004c) recommends that 15–25 strips be used for human studies. The amount of stratum corneum on each tape strip can be obtained by weighing (Pirot et al., 1998; Weigmann et al., 2003). Indirectly, it can be determined by measuring the amount of proteins on the tape (Chao & Nylander-French, 2004), by monitoring of transepidermal water loss (Weigmann et al., 2005), or spectrophotometrically by measuring light absorption of the proteins on the tape (Weigmann et al., 2003).

There are three different approaches in the methods that utilize the tape-stripping technique. The United States Food and Drug Administration (USFDA, 1998) has proposed a guideline for the determination of bioequivalence of topically applied products using a tape-stripping technique. The method is based on the determination of the total amount of drug in the collected strips in the stratum corneum during uptake and elimination phases. For drug uptake, the product is applied at multiple sites, and the stratum corneum samples are removed from each site just after removal of the applied drug at sequentially increasing times. To assess drug elimination, the drug is applied to multiple sites and maintained for a period of time. All the application sites are then cleaned, and the stratum corneum is removed at different times after cleaning. Bioequivalence is assessed based on the AUC. The results are plotted as the amount/surface area against time. The method was shown to be useful in determining the rate and extent of drug penetration into the stratum corneum (Shah et al., 1998; Weigmann et al., 2001; Pershing et al., 2002a,b, 2003). However, this method has not yet been sufficiently validated, and there has been some criticism of the method concerning its robustness, reliability, and reproducibility for bioequivalence testing. The USFDA withdrew the dermatopharmacokinetics (DPK) guidance in 2002, citing two principal concerns: 1) the adequacy of the method to assess the bioequivalence of topical dermatological drug products, and 2) the reproducibility of the method between laboratories (USFDA, 2001).

Another approach using the skin-stripping technique is based on the determination of the concentration profile of a chemical in the stratum corneum in relation to the relative stratum corneum depth. The depth of the stratum corneum for each strip can be estimated from the mass of the stratum corneum stripped off from each consecutive tape. The data on concentration–stratum corneum depth profile were fitted into a solution of Fick's second law of diffusion. From this, the partition coefficient of a chemical between the stratum corneum and a vehicle (K_m) and diffusivity (D) were derived, enabling deduction of the chemical permeability coefficient K_p (e.g. Pirot et al., 1998; Alberti et al., 2001; Reddy et al., 2002). However, this analysis assumes a profile consistent with a homogeneous membrane, and this is not always observed (Mueller et al., 2003).

Finally, tape-stripping studies also follow an approach in which the chemical is applied for a single exposure period and then the amount of chemical in collected tape strips is determined (e.g. Dupuis et al., 1984; Rougier et al., 1999; Chao & Nylander-French, 2004; Mattorano et al., 2004).

There are several problems encountered in the studies performing tape stripping. Some authors do not measure the actual depth of the stratum corneum but instead rely on the number of consecutive strips used, assuming regular stripping of stratum corneum. However, it has been shown that even in the case of very strict standardized protocols, the amount of stratum corneum on each tape strip varies considerably (Weigmann et al., 1999; Dickel et al., 2004). Furthermore, it has been shown that due to furrows in the stratum corneum, the amount of chemical measured in a particular strip comes from different layers, which might lead to misinterpretation of the results (van der Molen et al., 1997). For rapidly penetrating compounds, results from tape-stripping experiments can be affected significantly by chemical diffusion into the stratum corneum during the time required to apply and remove all of the tape strips (Reddy et al., 2002).

Because it can be used to test absorption in humans in vivo, tape stripping offers opportunities for studies that cannot be conducted readily in vitro or in laboratory animals. For example, diseased compared with healthy skin can be studied, as described by Jakasa et al. (2004a). In a tape-stripping study, the skin site of atopics that was not affected by disease showed higher stratum corneum penetration compared with healthy subjects. Furthermore, tape stripping can be used as a means of comparing human in vivo and in vitro data (e.g. Trebilcock et al., 1994; Pirot et al., 1998; Reddy et al., 2002).

7.3 Other methods

7.3.1 Whole-body autoradiography

Whole-body autoradiography is a useful technique used to determine the distribution of radiolabelled compounds in frozen cross-sections of the entire animal. This method has been shown to be a very useful tool for visualization of the radiolabelled chemical in all body tissues. By using microautoradiography, the distribution of a topically applied radiolabelled compound in specific areas of the skin can be determined (Lockley et al., 2004). In a study by Saleh et al. (1997), the distribution of [^{14}C]malathion, an organophosphorus pesticide, was investigated using electronic autoradiography of whole-body sections of treated rats after intravenous, oral, and dermal administration. Whereas the liver and kidney accumulated high levels of the chemical after intravenous administration, it was shown that the skin may act as a reservoir for the compound after dermal application.

The whole-body autoradiography technique is becoming more commonplace, although there are no guidelines to cover it.

7.3.2 Skin biopsy

A number of studies undertaken by Schaefer and colleagues (Kammerau et al., 1975; Zesch & Schaefer, 1975; Schaefer & Stuttgen, 1976; Kranz et al., 1977; Schaefer et al., 1977, 1978) have measured the dermal levels of various drugs in humans in vivo and in vitro. Much lower levels were found in vitro, demonstrating the role of blood flow in dermal absorption. Singh & Roberts (1994) used similar techniques in rats to show direct topical penetration of drugs into dermal and deeper tissue levels at early times after dosing. They also found that vasoconstriction increased dermal levels (Singh & Roberts, 1994). A number of authors have described the dermal concentration gradient by a dermal tissue diffusion–dermal blood flow clearance model (Gupta et al., 1995; Cross & Roberts, 1999; Kretsos et al., 2004; Kretsos & Kasting, 2005).

7.4 Factors affecting dermal absorption in vivo

7.4.1 Species, strain, and sex

The skin of rats, guinea-pigs, and rabbits is more permeable than that of humans, whereas the skin permeability of pigs and monkeys is more similar to that of humans (OECD, 2004b). Other possible animal models include the athymic (nude) rat skin flap model, hairless rats, hairless mice, and fuzzy rats (Klain & Reifenrath, 1991). In a comparative study involving several species, radiolabelled haloprogin, *N*-acetylcysteine, cortisone, testosterone, caffeine, and butter yellow dissolved in acetone were applied to the skin of rats, rabbits, minipigs, and humans (only haloprogin and *N*-acetylcysteine). The dose was 4 µg/cm^2 skin surface applied using a non-occlusive foam pad. The amount of radioactivity excreted in urine for 5 days following application of the test compound was used for quantifying skin absorption. The results obtained in this study indicated that dermal absorption decreases in the following order: rabbit, rat, pig, and human (see Figure 11) (Bartek et al., 1972).

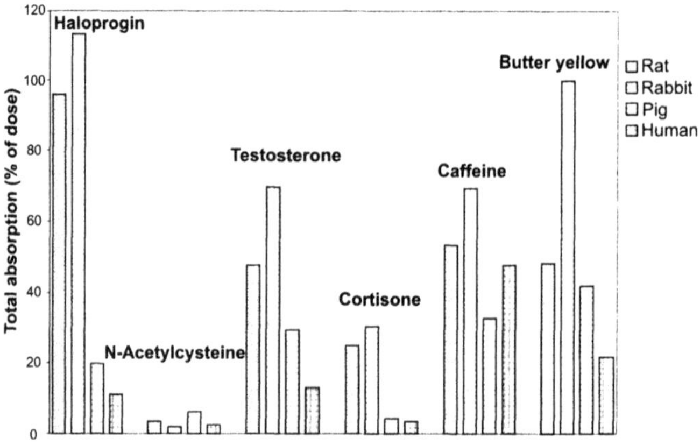

Fig. 11. Total absorption of different compounds in different species (adapted from Bartek et al., 1972).

7.4.2 Age

In a comparative study with human volunteers, Roskos et al. (1989) demonstrated that age can affect dermal absorption. Permeation of hydrocortisone, benzoic acid, acetylsalicylic acid, and caffeine was significantly lower in aged subjects, whereas the absorption of testosterone and estradiol was similar in young and aged subjects. An explanation might be that the diminished surface lipid content and reduced hydration of "old" skin imply a diminished dissolution medium for compounds administered topically, which reduces the uptake of somewhat hydrophilic compounds especially. In contrast, highly lipid-soluble chemicals such as testosterone and estrogen may still be able to dissolve readily into the stratum corneum, even when the available lipid medium is reduced (Roskos et al., 1989).

7.4.3 Anatomical site

The percutaneous absorption of acetylsalicylic acid, benzoic acid, caffeine, and benzoic acid sodium salt (radiolabelled) was measured in male Caucasians on four body sites (arm, abdomen, postauricular, forehead), using the tape-stripping method. Skin penetration, as indicated by the amount of chemical in the stratum corneum, was ranked as follows: arm $\leq$ abdomen $\leq$ postauricular $\leq$ forehead. It is noteworthy that whatever the compound applied, the forehead was about twice as permeable as the arm or the abdomen (Rougier et al., 1987, 1999).

Absorption of radiolabelled cortisol through various anatomical sites after topical application of hydrocortisone in acetone to male volunteers (13 cm^2 skin surface) was studied by analysing the urine for a total of 5 days. The absorption through the forearm of each volunteer served as control. The results are shown in Figure 12. A number of other studies are summarized in Roberts & Walters (1998).

These and similar data on hydrocortisone and pesticides were combined to construct penetration indices for five anatomical sites, as shown in Table 5 (Wester & Maibach, 1999a).

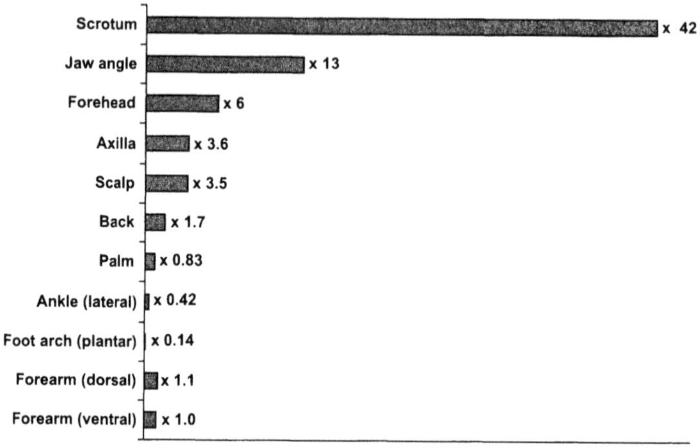

Fig. 12. Hydrocortisone absorption — effect of anatomical region (adapted from Feldmann & Maibach, 1967).

Table 5. Penetration indices for different anatomical sites

Site	Penetration index based on	
	Hydrocortisone data	Pesticide data
Genitals	40	12
Arms	1	1
Legs	0.5	1
Trunk	2.5	3
Head	5	4

Although all authors agree on the importance of anatomical location in percutaneous absorption, the reviews on this topic give contradictory explanations. Factors that influence regional differences in skin permeability include different thicknesses and composition of the stratum corneum in different anatomical locations, size and number of follicles, sebum composition, etc. (Scheuplein & Blank, 1971; Idson, 1975; Roberts et al., 1982; Barry, 1983). A further explanation may be the closeness of capillaries to the surface of the skin in certain regions of the body. This effect may promote resorption and may explain high percutaneous penetration in the postauricular area found for benzoic acid, benzoic acid sodium salt, and acetylsalicylic acid (Rougier et al., 1999).

7.4.4 Type of application and vehicle

Applied vehicles have the potential to either increase or decrease the solubility and/or diffusion of a compound in the horny layer and, thereby, to increase or decrease penetration.

The penetration of benzoic acid is enhanced by increasing the water content of the vehicles, whatever the organic phase (Rougier et al., 1999). The influence of nine vehicles on the in vivo percutaneous absorption of radiolabelled benzoic acid was studied in the hairless rat, by assessing total percutaneous absorption and stratum corneum reservoir (stripping method) (Rougier et al., 1999). Each vehicle (propylene glycol/triton X-100 90:10, glycerol/triton X-100 90:10, ethylene glycol/triton X-100 90:10, ethylene glycol/triton X-100 90:10/water 40:60, propylene glycol/triton X-100 90:10/water 40:60, ethanol/water 95:5, methanol/water 40:60, ethanol/water 60:40, ethanol/water 40:60), containing 200 nmol of benzoic acid, was applied to 1 cm^2 of dorsal skin during 30 min. Although the vehicles used were simple in composition, the total amount of benzoic acid that penetrated over 4 days varied by a factor of 50. This influence of the presence of water on the dermal absorption was also reported in volunteers using 2-butoxyethanol. The percutaneous absorption of the test substance from aqueous solution increased markedly when compared with neat 2-butoxyethanol. As little as 10% water in 2-butoxyethanol produced approximately a 4-fold increase in the permeation rates (Jakasa et al., 2004b). Similar results were obtained in rats (EDETOX, 2004; see Appendix 2). Contrary to this, dermal penetration of neat chloroform was higher than that of aqueous solutions containing chloroform (Islam et al., 1999); however, this was probably due to damage of the skin caused by neat solvent.

White spirit enhanced the penetration of lindane compared with an acetone vehicle (Dick et al., 1997a). For studies on the influence of vehicles in in vitro studies, see section 6.5.5.

7.4.5 *Temperature and humidity conditions*

Increased percutaneous absorption rates were seen for 2-butoxyethanol vapours with raised temperature and humidity conditions (Johanson & Boman, 1991; Jones et al., 2003). The mean "baseline" (25 °C, 40% relative humidity, shorts and T-shirts) percentage of dermal absorption was 11% (range 9–14%) of the "whole-body" burden. For each subsequent exposure, a single parameter was changed: humidity (60%, 65%), temperature (20 °C, 30 °C), or clothing (minimal or overalls). At 30 °C, the percentage of dermal absorption was significantly increased, with a mean of 14% (range 12–15%). Increasing the humidity increased the percentage of dermal absorption, although not significantly. Clothing also had little effect on the percentage of dermal absorption. In an "industrial" scenario (30 °C, 60–65% relative humidity, overalls) that might be encountered in a tank cleaning or similar operation, skin absorption was significantly increased (mean of 39%) when compared with the baseline dermal study (Jones et al., 2003).

The absorption of transdermally delivered nicotine to human volunteers increased after they stayed in a sauna bath (mean temperature 82 °C, 28% humidity) for three 10-min periods separated by two 5-min breaks, compared with measurements taken in a previous control session (without sauna) (Vanakoski et al., 1996).

8. COMPARATIVE STUDIES

8.1 Comparison between in vitro and in vivo skin absorption results

Many studies have compared in vitro and in vivo percutaneous absorption (Table 6). In general, they verify the premise that properly conducted in vitro measurements can be used to predict in vivo absorption. The basis of OECD Test Guideline 428 (OECD, 2004c) is that in vitro studies can predict in vivo absorption when the correct methodology for both tests is used.

Table 6. Some comparative studies on dermal absorption in vitro and in vivo

Compounds	Species	Lipophilicity/polarity	References
12 organic compounds	Human	Mixed polarity	Franz (1975, 1978)
Benzoic acid, acetylsalicylic acid, urea, and caffeine	Rat	Generally polar	Bronaugh et al. (1982)
Nitroaromatic compounds	Monkey, human	Mixed polarity	Bronaugh & Maibach (1985)
Benzoic acid, caffeine, and testosterone	Human	Mixed polarity	Bronaugh & Franz (1986)
Anthracene	Rat	Lipophilic	Yang et al. (1986a)
Benzo[*a*]pyrene	Rat	Lipophilic	Yang et al. (1986b)
Cypermethrin (pesticide)	Rat	Lipophilic	Scott & Ramsey (1987)
5 pesticides	Mouse	Lipophilic and hydrophilic	Grissom et al. (1987)
Phenoxy herbicides 2,4-D, 2,4-D amine	Rat, rabbit, rhesus monkey, human	Mixed polarity	Moody et al. (1990)
Benzyl acetate	Rat	Lipophilic	Hotchkiss et al. (1990)
Phenanthrene	Guinea-pig	Lipophilic	Ng et al. (1991)

Table 6 (Contd)

Compounds	Species	Lipophilicity/polarity	References
Tritiated water, ethanol, mannitol, paraquat	Rat, marmoset, human	Hydrophilic	Scott et al. (1991a)
8 pesticides (identity not given)	Rat	Mixed polarity	Scott et al. (1992)
Pyrene, benzo[*a*]pyrene, di(2-ethylhexyl)-phthalate	Guinea-pig	Lipophilic	Ng et al. (1992)
Fluazifop-butyl	Rat, human	Lipophilic	Ramsey et al. (1992, 1994)
Nitroglycerine	Human	Lipophilic	Hadgraft et al. (1993)
Hair dyes	Rat, pig	Mixed polarity	Beck et al. (1994)
Vanilloids	Rat	Lipophilic	Kasting et al. (1997)
Lindane	Human	Lipophilic	Dick et al. (1997a,b)
Methyl salicylate	Human	Lipophilic	Cross et al. (1998)
Propoxur	Rat, human	Hydrophilic	van de Sandt et al. (2000)
Ortho-Phenyl-phenol	Rat, human	Lipophilic	Cnubben et al. (2002)
2-Butoxyethanol	Human	Hydrophilic	Jakasa et al. (2004b)
14 pesticides	Rat	Mixed polarity	van Ravenzwaay & Leibold (2004)

There are some exceptions; for example, for radiolabelled 2-nitro-*p*-phenylenediamine, 4-amino-2-nitrophenol, nitrobenzene, *p*-nitroaniline, and 2,4-dinitrochlorobenzene (4 μg/cm^2, acetone, 24 h), the absorption in monkeys was slightly less in vitro than in vivo, but the values were not significantly different (Bronaugh & Maibach, 1985). Another example was the volatile compound nitrobenzene, where human data indicated significantly higher percutaneous absorption in vivo compared with in vitro (Bronaugh & Maibach, 1985).

A comparison of the in vitro and in vivo percutaneous absorption of caffeine and testosterone in three vehicles (petrolatum, ethylene glycol gel, and water gel) revealed no significant differences between most values. However, there was a trend towards lower penetration in the in vitro system (Bronaugh & Franz, 1986). In vitro absorption utilizing flow-through diffusion methodology with human cadaver skin and human plasma receptor fluid gave a per cent dose absorbed similar to that in in vivo human volunteer studies for the pesticide isofenphos (Wester et al., 1992).

The in vitro and in vivo absorption and metabolism of pyrene, benzo[*a*]pyrene, and di(2-ethylhexyl)phthalate were investigated in hairless guinea-pig. The in vitro method, which involved the use of flow-through diffusion cells and HEPES-buffered Hanks' balanced salt solution containing 4% bovine serum albumin as perfusate, was shown to be a suitable system for predicting in vivo absorption of these lipophilic compounds (Ng et al., 1992).

The dermal absorption of [^{14}C]benzo[*a*]pyrene was studied in vitro in different species (rat, hairless guinea-pig, 50- and 32-year-old human volunteers) and in vivo in rat and hairless guinea-pig. The total percentage of [^{14}C]benzo[*a*]pyrene absorbed in vitro was consistent with that absorbed in vivo, both demonstrating that benzo[*a*]pyrene was well absorbed through skin (Moody et al., 1995).

Many of the in vitro/in vivo (human) comparisons have been made with pesticides, including cypermethrin (Scott & Ramsey, 1987) and fluazifop-butyl (Ramsey et al., 1994). In addition, comparative studies in rats have shown the predictive ability of the in vitro method (Scott et al., 1992; van Ravenzwaay & Leibold, 2004).

Beck et al. (1994) compared in vivo and in vitro data on dermal absorption of hair dyes in studies with rats and pigs. The data were from two laboratories; the studies had been performed under similar conditions, but in general were spaced by several years, were performed by different persons, and used different chamber systems. The authors found that, despite these differences, the comparisons were good between in vivo and in vitro results. Dick et al. (1997a,b) investigated the dermal absorption of lindane from acetone and a white spirit–based formulation in in vitro and in vivo studies using human volunteers. The in vitro studies predicted the 40-fold difference in absorption between the two applications observed in the volunteers.

Jung et al. (2003) carried out in vitro and in vivo percutaneous studies with catechol. Total in vitro skin penetration was 1.4-fold higher than in vivo skin penetration. However, there were differences in conditions (e.g. the dorsal skin temperature of fuzzy rat was 35 °C, and the in vitro studies were carried out at 32 °C). There were low recovery rates in the in vivo study compared with the in vitro study.

In a study on the pesticide propoxur, the experimental conditions were standardized with respect to dose, vehicle, and exposure duration (van de Sandt et al., 2000). In vivo studies were performed in rats and human volunteers, while in vitro experiments were carried out in static diffusion cells using viable skin membranes (rat and human), non-viable epidermal membranes (rat and human), and a perfused pig ear model. In vivo and in vitro absorption were compared on the basis of the absorbed dose after 4 and 24 h, the maximum flux, the lag time, and the potential absorbed dose.

In human volunteers, it was found that approximately 6% of the applied dose (150 μg/cm^2) was excreted via the urine (as the metabolite 2-isopropoxyphenol) after 24 h, while the potentially absorbed dose (amount applied minus amount washed off) was 23 μg/cm^2. In rats, these values were 21% and 88 μg/cm^2, respectively. Data obtained in vitro were almost always higher than those obtained in human volunteers. The potentially absorbed dose seemed to give the best prediction of human in vivo percutaneous absorption. The absorbed dose and the maximum flux in viable full-thickness skin membranes corresponded well with the human in vivo situation (maximum overestimation 3-fold); epidermal membranes overestimated the human in vivo data by up to a factor of 8 (van de Sandt et al., 2000).

The same group carried out a second study (Cnubben et al., 2002) assessing the percutaneous penetration of the fungicide *ortho*-phenylphenol using various in vitro approaches — static diffusion cells with viable full-thickness skin membranes of rats and humans, non-viable epidermal membranes of rats and humans, and a perfused pig ear model — and compared the results with respective in vivo rat and human volunteer data using standardized conditions (Figure 13). In viable full-thickness skin membranes, the amount systemically available and the potentially absorbed dose correlated reasonably well with the human in vivo situation. In contrast, the maximum flux considerably underestimated the human in vivo situation. The results obtained with epidermal membranes again overestimated human in vivo absorption data (Cnubben et al., 2002).

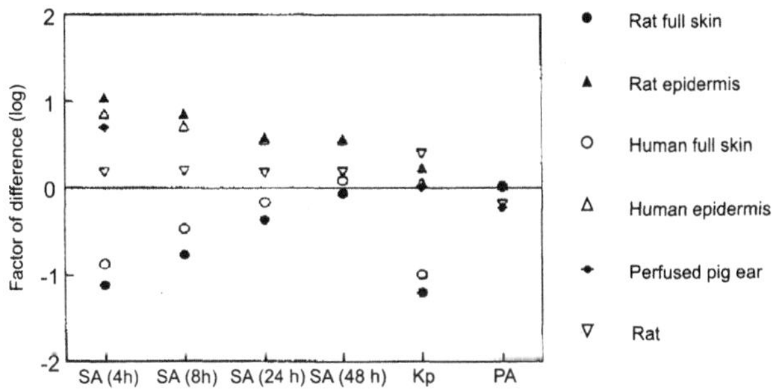

Fig. 13. Factor of difference; compared with human volunteer data between in vitro and in vivo skin absorption of [^{14}C]*ortho*-phenylphenol based on the systemically available amount (SA) at 4, 8, 24, and 48 h after a 4-h exposure period of 120 µg/cm^2, the permeability coefficient (K_p), and the potentially absorbed dose (PA) (from Cnubben et al., 2002). [Reprinted from Regulatory Toxicology and Pharmacology, Vol. 35, No. 1, N.H. Cnubben et al., Comparative in vitro–in vivo percutaneous penetration of the fungicide *ortho*-phenylphenol, Pages 198–208, Copyright (2002), with permission from Elsevier]

The extent of skin first-pass metabolism (Roberts & Walters, 1998) can also vary between in vitro and in vivo studies (see chapter 5). In general, the skin first-pass metabolism is more extensive in vivo than in vitro, as illustrated by methyl salicylate (Cross et al., 1998). Hence, failure to recognize this first-pass effect in in vitro studies can lead to an overestimate of the systemic exposure after topical application in vivo.

In the EDETOX (undated) project, dermal absorption studies in human volunteers were conducted in parallel with in vitro predictions with human skin using the same dose, vehicle, and application time for 50% 2-butoxyethanol/water (Wilkinson & Williams, 2002;

Jakasa et al., 2004b). There was a close relationship between absorption rate determined in vitro and that determined from in vivo data (2.0 μg/cm^2 per hour in vitro with dermatomed skin compared with 2.7 μg/cm^2 per hour determined from in vivo data).

There was also a good relationship between in vivo and in vitro data for 50% butoxyethanol in the rat (2.0 μg/cm^2 per hour compared with 1.3 μg/cm^2 per hour). A similar relationship was also observed for the rat for di(2-ethylhexyl)phthalate, pyrene, and benzo[*a*]pyrene, although the in vivo data were slightly underestimated.

Although the above studies show more the exceptions to the observation of a good correlation between in vitro and in vivo data, there are many examples of studies in which in vitro and in vivo data correlated well. The reason for the lack of correlation may be that the experimental conditions may not have been correctly controlled in the above examples, as they were conducted prior to the adoption of OECD Test Guideline 428 (OECD, 2004c).

8.2 Inter- and intralaboratory variation in in vitro percutaneous absorption methodology

As in vitro measurements of skin absorption are an increasingly important aspect of regulatory studies, potential sources of inter- and intralaboratory variations have to be investigated. Much effort has been expended in comparing the different diffusion cells used to measure percutaneous penetration, and it is generally accepted that most diffusion cell systems provide comparable measurements of skin absorption rates for a range of penetrants. It is well documented that there is a large (natural) variation in skin permeability (Southwell et al., 1984). However, in addition to the known factors influencing percutaneous penetration (see Table 1 in chapter 2), which have been discussed in other parts of this document, there is a likelihood of inter- and intralaboratory variation. A few studies have investigated this.

The in vitro absorption of benzoic acid, caffeine, and testosterone — representing a range of different physicochemical properties — through human skin (nine laboratories) and rat skin (one laboratory) was determined (van de Sandt et al., 2004). All laboratories performed their studies according to detailed protocols (dose, exposure time, vehicle, receptor fluid, preparation of membranes, analysis), and each laboratory performed at least three independent experiments (containing at least 5–7 replicates per experiment) for each test chemical. The ranking of dermal absorption of all chemicals was the same for all participating laboratories. There was variability between laboratories with respect to the total absorption data (benzoic acid 22.5%; caffeine 40.9%; testosterone 64.3%; all percentages are coefficients of variation over six laboratories), most likely due, to a large extent, to interindividual variability in absorption between samples of human skin and differences in skin site and source. The intralaboratory variation was influenced by the skin itself. Skin thickness only slightly influenced the absorption of benzoic acid and caffeine; however, the maximum absorption rate of the most lipophilic compound, testosterone, was clearly higher in the laboratories using thin, dermatomed skin membranes (van de Sandt et al., 2004).

In an international multicentre study involving 18 laboratories, interlaboratory and intralaboratory variations in diffusion cell measurements were determined using a silicon rubber membrane, thereby excluding skin variability (Chilcott et al., 2005). The study was performed using a standard penetrant, methyl paraben, and an appropriate standard protocol. "Standardized" calculations of methyl paraben flux were determined by a central laboratory from the data submitted by each laboratory. The coefficient of variation between laboratories was approximately 35%. There was a 4-fold difference between the lowest and highest average flux values and a 6-fold difference between the lowest and highest individual flux values. Intralaboratory variation was lower, averaging 10% for five individuals using the same equipment within a single laboratory.

Vecchia & Bunge (2003a) compared quality-controlled measurements for human skin permeability coefficients from multiple laboratories. The variation was between 1 and 2 orders of magnitude. A similar degree of variability has been shown for maximum flux (Magnusson et al., 2004a).

These variations reinforce the need to conduct carefully controlled in vitro and in vivo dermal absorption studies.

9. DATA COLLECTIONS

Over the decades, a large number of data have been generated on the percutaneous penetration of a wide range of chemicals, including pesticides, cosmetics, and pharmaceuticals. Studies have included work on human volunteers and in vivo studies using animal models (see chapter 7) and in vitro studies on excised human, rodent, pig, guinea-pig, and, more recently, synthetic skin (see chapter 6). There has, until recently (OECD, 2004a,b,c), been no agreed standard procedure for measuring dermal absorption. There are numerous factors that can influence dermal penetration values, such as species variation, application site, dosing regime, occlusion, sex, and age, as well as interlaboratory and intralaboratory variations (see Table 1 in chapter 2).

While many of these studies on percutaneous penetration are unpublished (being company or governmental property), there are a number of studies in the open literature. There have been many different compilations of data (e.g. Flynn, 1985; Johnson et al., 1995; Wilschut et al., 1995; Patel et al., 2002; Vecchia & Bunge, 2003a; USEPA, 2004b). Under the auspices of the EDETOX project, a database has been compiled giving details of studies on percutaneous penetration. This database is freely available on the EDETOX web site. Therefore, in the present document, it was not attempted to mention every study, as these can be found easily in this EDETOX database (http://www.ncl.ac.uk/edetox).

9.1 Data sets from homologous or closely related molecules

As well as studies on single compounds, several investigators determined permeability data from homologous or closely related series of molecules (see Table 7). These data have been used for modelling skin permeability in these series (Marzulli et al., 1965; Scheuplein & Blank, 1971; Idson, 1975; Roberts et al., 1977; Wester & Maibach, 1985; Idson & Behl, 1987; Ridout & Guy, 1988; Ridout et al., 1992). An overview of several of the combined data sets is provided by Vecchia & Bunge (2003a,c). There has been discussion about the quality of the steroid data from Scheuplein et al. (1969) (Moss & Cronin, 2002; Moss et al., 2002).

Table 7. Permeability data sets for some homologous or closely related series of molecules

Molecules	References
n-Alkanols	Scheuplein & Blank (1971, 1973); Flynn & Yalkowsky (1972); Wiechers (1989)
Ethyl ether, 2-butanone, 1-butanol, 2-ethoxyethanol, 2,3-butanediol	Blank et al. (1967)
Steroids	Scheuplein et al. (1969)
Hydrocortisone-21 esters (and 5'-vidarabine esters)	Flynn (1985)
Phenolic compounds	Roberts et al. (1977)
Glycol ethers	Dugard et al. (1984)
8 salicylates and 10 non-steroidal anti-inflammatory drugs in humans	Yano et al. (1986)
Hair dyes	Bronaugh & Congdon (1984)
Metals	Hostynek (2003)
Aromatic amines	Levillain et al. (1998)
Para-substituted phenols	Hinz et al. (1991)
PAHs	Roy et al. (1998)

9.2 Flynn data set

A milestone in the development of percutaneous absorption prediction was the publication of what is now known as the Flynn data set. This is a publication of 97 permeability coefficients for 94 compounds in vitro through human skin and for toluene, ethyl benzene, and styrene in vivo in humans (Flynn, 1990) and was for over a decade the largest database of skin permeability values. However, this is a compilation of 15 different literature sources (some of these are given in Table 7), with the inherent disadvantage of having a high degree of variability due to interlaboratory and intralaboratory error as well as variation due to the skin being from different sources and locations in the body (Moss et al., 2002). Based on this data set, Flynn and several others have proposed a number of algorithms to predict skin permeability (see chapter 10 on QSARs).

9.3 Expanded permeability coefficient data sets

For modelling studies, a number of data sets were compiled from various earlier publications. For example, in the study by Wilschut et al. (1995), data were given on 123 measured permeability coefficients of 99 different chemicals; Vecchia & Bunge (2003a) presented a sizeable and diverse data set of 170 measurements for 127 compounds covering relative molecular weights from 18 to 584 and log K_{ow} values from −3.1 to 4.6; Patel et al. (2002) collected a comprehensive data set containing 186 permeability coefficients for some 158 structurally diverse compounds (from human in vitro skin data) (see also chapter 10).

Further, there are repositories of data kept by industry and regulatory bodies (e.g. pesticide data sets, held by the United States Environmental Protection Agency [USEPA], of almost 300 dermal absorption studies of more than 160 different pesticides; Reddy & Bunge, 2002; Jones et al., 2004).

9.4 EDETOX database

The EDETOX database was generated within the EDETOX project, a multipartner project funded under the European Union's (EU) Framework V Programme (EDETOX, 2004, undated; see also section A2.3 in Appendix A). The purpose of the database was to bring together in vivo and in vitro percutaneous absorption and distribution data from all available sources, together with the physicochemical data for each chemical of interest (Soyei & Williams, 2004). The database contains over 4800 studies for 320 chemicals.

Studies entering the database were assessed as to whether they satisfied the following EDETOX criteria:

- chemical concentration (of chemical applied);
- dose volume (volume of chemical applied to skin);
- loading (amount of chemical added per unit area);
- area (area of skin to which the chemical was applied);
- vehicle (application medium);
- species (species of animal used in the study);
- exposure time (length of time the chemical was left on the skin);

- analytical method (method by which the results were determined);
- receptor fluid (medium that bathes the underside of the skin); and
- temperature (temperature of the receptor fluid/skin/water bath during in vitro experiments).

Initially, it was intended to include only papers that satisfied the EDETOX criteria. However, very few did. Therefore, all papers were entered, but those not fitting the criteria (well over 50%) were highlighted as such (Soyei & Williams, 2004). The database can be accessed at http://www.ncl.ac.uk/edetox (EDETOX, undated).

9.5 Maximum flux databases

There appear to be only a limited number of maximum flux databases for solutes in human skin. Early databases for alcohols and phenolic compounds were described by Scheuplein & Blank (1973) and Roberts et al. (1977). Perhaps the first database for a range of heterogeneous compounds from one vehicle (propylene glycol) was described by Kasting et al. (1987). A maximum flux database for 278 compounds has recently been described and is available as supplemental material from the *Journal of Investigative Dermatology* (online) at http://www.nature.com/jid/journal/v122/n4/suppinfo/5602287s1.html?url=/jid/journal/v122/n4/full/5602287a.html. The criteria for inclusion of these compounds are included in the accompanying paper (Magnusson et al., 2004a).

10. ESTIMATION/PREDICTION OF DERMAL PENETRATION

There has been much interest in the potential to predict dermal absorption and avoid unnecessary and costly in vitro and in vivo testing. This is partly due to ethical difficulties with respect to human and laboratory animal experiments and partly due to economic and time considerations as a result of increasing legislation in the risk assessment of industrial chemicals (e.g. proposed new European chemicals strategy: Registration, Evaluation, Authorisation and Restriction of Chemicals, or REACH) (see also Jones et al., 2004).

QSARs are generally used to relate properties of chemicals to biological effects or transport properties and are an observation of the association between an outcome and the properties likely to affect that outcome. A QSAR provides predictions of coefficients needed to estimate absorption for untested chemicals. It is not an expression of theoretical physical relationships (e.g. mass balance) and is therefore complementary to mathematical transport models describing dermal absorption. Mathematical models simulate the sequence of partition and transport processes involved in dermal absorption (see chapter 4) and can predict the extent and rate of chemical permeation through the skin (Fitzpatrick et al., 2004). Mathematical modelling plays a key role in linking permeability coefficient data obtained from tests under steady-state conditions (i.e. infinite dose) to absorption estimates for finite dose applications that are more typical of occupational exposure (i.e. non-steady-state conditions) (Jones et al., 2004). However, it should be noted that, in the simplest case, a parameter additional to the permeability coefficient K_p (i.e. the partition coefficient K_m) is needed to model absorption from finite doses (Scheuplein & Ross, 1974). In reality, the nature of the finite dose, interfacial resistances, and the receptor sampling conditions will also affect model estimations (Anissimov & Roberts, 2001).

10.1 QSAR analysis

QSARs, when applied to estimating dermal permeability coefficients, are sometimes known as quantitative structure–permeability relationships (QSPeRs or QSPRs). Recent overviews of QSPeRs for permeation into human skin from water are given by Moss et al. (2002), Vecchia & Bunge (2003a,b), Walker et al. (2003), Fitzpatrick et al. (2004), and Geinoz et al. (2004).

10.1.1 Prerequisites for QSPeR analysis

Ideally, the QSPeRs are related to the mechanism of dermal penetration, which depends on the structure of the skin (see chapter 3). Considering the passage of a chemical through the skin from water, the stratum corneum is essentially a tightly bound lipophilic layer, which interfaces with an aqueous vehicle. Therefore, descriptors of hydrophobicity, molecular size, and possibly hydrogen bonding (which may describe non-covalent interactions with skin proteins) are of importance for the development of QSARs (Moss et al., 2002).

QSPeRs are statistically derived linear and non-linear relationships between the steady-state permeability of a compound, usually measured from water, and various physicochemical descriptors and/or structural properties of the molecule. QSPeRs often are derived using parameters that themselves are calculated from QSARs. For example, the octanol/water partition coefficient K_{ow} has often been used as an input parameter to QSPeR equations. While K_{ow} has been measured for some chemicals, for others a QSAR prediction is used, and these values will reflect the predictive limitations of the QSAR, particularly when it is used outside its predictive domain. Various software programs can provide differing estimates for K_{ow} and solute solubility.

The statistical nature of such QSARs means that the more data used to derive a relationship, the more reliable the QSAR is likely to be for predictive purposes, assuming that the relationship is acceptable from a statistical point of view and that the data themselves are deemed to be sufficiently varied and of satisfactory quality. For a QSPeR, the data (observed permeation) should be consistent, produced from standardized experimental procedures, and obtained for a set of chemicals that cover the domain of relevant chemical properties (Jones et al., 2004).

The dermal absorption measurement that has been most widely used in QSAR modelling is the permeability coefficient K_p, because it characterizes the steady-state permeation rate of a chemical from a specific vehicle through a given membrane. Although K_p is not directly suitable for application in risk assessment, it can be used in conjunction with measured (or estimated) solubility in the same vehicle as was used for the K_p measurement (usually water) to predict a maximum flux through the skin (Jones et al., 2004). Also, as stated above, it can be combined in mathematical models with partition coefficient values for the skin (either from measurements or from QSAR predictions) to estimate non-steady-state or finite dose absorption.

The permeability coefficient K_p of a substance through the stratum corneum is given by:

$$K_p = K_m \cdot D / h \qquad \text{[Equation 4 in chapter 4]}$$

where h is the apparent thickness of the stratum corneum, D is the effective permeant diffusivity in the stratum corneum, and K_m is the partition coefficient between the stratum corneum and the vehicle. The partition coefficient from an aqueous vehicle, K_m, has been shown to be related to K_{ow} (Cleek & Bunge, 1993; Roberts et al., 1996; Vecchia & Bunge, 2003c). In reality, the stratum corneum is heterogeneous, and the differential partitioning into protein and lipid components (Raykar et al., 1988) should be recognized, as this better determines solute permeation through the stratum corneum (Anderson & Raykar, 1989; Nitsche et al., 2006; Wang et al., 2006).

10.1.2 Historical overview

10.1.2.1 QSPeRs for skin permeability prior to the 1990s

The majority of these older studies were based on the analysis of homologous, or closely related, series of molecules, and often only a relatively small number of compounds were assessed (see chapter 9). Many of these studies revealed that skin permeability increased in a linear relationship with hydrophobicity (Scheuplein & Blank, 1971; Roberts et al., 1977). Some studies also reported a parabolic relationship with hydrophobicity, particularly if there was a selection of compounds that included those that were highly hydrophobic (Scheuplein & Blank, 1971). However, each model existed in isolation for a particular class or series of compounds. Further, as a consequence, there was co-linearity between the descriptors for a congeneric series — for example, hydrophobicity and molecular size — so that it is not possible to distinguish between the effects of these two factors on the permeability of large hydrophobic molecules (Moss et al., 2002).

10.1.2.2 *The Flynn (1990) data set and subsequent analyses*

Flynn (1990) proposed a number of algorithms to predict K_p, which stated that very hydrophilic and very hydrophobic compounds had low and high skin permeability, respectively, and that different K_{ow}-dependent QSARs could be used to predict skin permeability for high and low molecular weight compounds. Potts & Guy (1992) demonstrated the use of log K_{ow} in combination with either molecular weight (MW) or molecular volume to predict K_p data (in units of cm/h) collected by Flynn (1990):

$$\text{Log } K_p = 0.71 \log K_{ow} - 0.0061 \text{ MW} - 2.44 \qquad \text{[Equation 6]}$$
$$n = 93;\ r^2 = 0.67;\ s \text{ not reported};\ F \text{ not reported}$$

where n is the number of observations or number of compounds, r is the correlation coefficient, s is the standard error of the estimate, and F is Fisher's statistic.

Potts & Guy (1992) did not perform a full statistical analysis on the data set. Although both descriptors used in the above equation are statistically significant, the statistical fit to Equation 6 is comparatively poor (Moss et al., 2002). Potts & Guy (1992) did observe that up to a 30% variability in the experimental data was to be expected; however, they did not investigate the relationship for outliers or other statistical anomalies.

The publication of Flynn's (1990) large heterogeneous data set was a significant milestone and was subsequently the basis for several analyses and publications (see Table 8 and detailed discussion in Moss et al., 2002).

Table 8. A selection of recent QSPeR models illustrating sample size (number of compounds), correlation coefficient (r^2), and the source of the data used[a]

Model	n	r^2	Experimental data source
Flynn (1990)	95	–	Flynn (1990)
Potts & Guy (1992)	93	0.67	Flynn (1990)
Lien & Gao (1995)	22	0.96	Flynn (1990)
Barratt (1995a)	60	0.90	Flynn (1990)
Potts & Guy (1995)	37	0.94	Flynn (1990)
Abraham et al. (1995)	46	0.96	Flynn (1990)
Kirchner et al. (1997)	114	0.32	Flynn (1990) + Health Canada
Hostynek & Magee (1997)	20	0.80	Miscellaneous
Roy et al. (1998)	60	0.64	Roy et al. (1998)
Abraham et al. (1999)	53	0.96	Flynn (1990)
Gute et al. (1999)	60	0.67	Roy et al. (1998)
Cronin et al. (1999)	107	0.86	Flynn (1990) + Health Canada
Dearden et al. (2000)	91	0.83	Flynn (1990)
Patel et al. (2002)	143	0.90	Flynn (1990), Wilschut et al. (1995)
Vecchia & Bunge (2003a)	127	0.55	Flynn (1990) + miscellaneous

[a] From Fitzpatrick et al. (2004) and Vecchia & Bunge (2003a).

Reviews of modelling the skin permeability of homologous, or closely related, compounds are given by Scheuplein & Blank (1971), Idson (1975), Wester & Maibach (1985), Idson & Behl (1987), Ridout & Guy (1988), and Ridout et al. (1992). USEPA (1992) and USEPA (2004b) present a slightly modified version of the Potts & Guy (1992) correlation, which includes an adjustment for the transport resistance through the viable epidermis, as proposed by Cleek & Bunge (1993). USEPA (2004b) also presents the effective prediction domain for this correlation — i.e. the range of K_{ow} values and molecular weights for which this equation is valid (see Exhibit A-1 of that document).

A larger database of 114 skin permeability values was prepared by Kirchner et al. (1997) from the Flynn (1990) data set (51 chemicals), together with additional data from regulatory reports from Health Canada. However, data for 56 of the additional 63 chemicals were calculated using Equation 6 and were not experimental data (Poda et al., 2001; Frasch & Landsittel, 2002; Walker et al., 2003). Not realizing this, Cronin et al. (1999) analysed the Kirchner et al. (1997) database. After removing seven significant outliers (large compounds, such as estriol, atropine, hydrocortisone, etorphine, and digitoxin, as well as compounds with more than 10 sites to accept or donate a hydrogen bond), they analysed the database against a wide variety of QSAR parameters, including those for hydrogen bonding and other molecular properties. Not surprisingly, given the origins of nearly half of the data, the equation they derived, shown below, was similar to Equation 4:

$$\text{Log } K_p = 0.77 \log K_{ow} - 0.0103 \text{ MW} - 2.33 \qquad \text{[Equation 7]}$$
$$n = 107; r^2 = 0.86; s = 0.39; F = 317$$

Because it is based on a number of calculated rather than experimental data, Equation 7 should not be used (Frasch & Landsittel, 2002).

The problem of identifying and dealing with outliers is a controversial issue. From the various studies (Pugh & Hadgraft, 1994; Barratt, 1995a; Cronin et al., 1999), some compounds are found consistently as outliers. Reinvestigation of some of the values by Moss et al. (2002) and Moss & Cronin (2002) — e.g. permeability coefficients for steroids from Scheuplein et al. (1969) compared with measurements from Johnson et al. (1995); and permeability coefficients for diclofenac, naproxen, atropine, and nicotine compared with measurements from Degim et al. (1998) — showed that at least some of the data in the Flynn (1990) data set may have considerable error associated with them. This finding justified the exclusion of these compounds, for example, by Cronin et al. (1999), to produce a statistically valid model. This issue, in particular concerning steroid permeabilities, is extensively discussed in Moss et al. (2002).

Patel et al. (2002) collected a comprehensive data set containing 186 permeability coefficients for some 158 structurally diverse compounds from human in vitro skin data from Flynn (1990) and Wilschut et al. (1995). They removed some compounds (atropine, diclofenac, naproxen, nicotine) that were considered as outliers from the data set and developed a QSPeR that gave a value of $r^2 = 0.90$ for the remaining 143 compounds:

$$\text{Log } K_p = 0.652 \log K_{ow} - 0.00603 \text{ MW} - 6.23 \text{ ABSQon} - 0.313 \text{ SsssCH} - 2.30 \qquad \text{[Equation 8]}$$

where ABSQon is the sum of absolute charges on oxygen and nitrogen atoms and SsssCH is the sum of E-state indices for all methyl groups.

The authors also fitted these data with a QSPeR of the general form:

$$\text{Log } K_p = a \log K_{ow} - b(\text{molecular size}) + c \qquad \text{[Equation 9]}$$

Although calculated estimates of molecular volume have previously been shown to be better than molecular weight for the prediction of skin permeation (Barratt, 1995a; Potts & Guy, 1995), Patel et al. (2002) found molecular weight to be a better predictive model; it also has the advantage that it is an easier descriptor to obtain and apply. However, it must be recognized that the data set they examined is dominated by hydrocarbons with relatively constant values in the ratio of molecular volume to molecular weight. For compounds with ratios of molecular volume to molecular weight that deviate from the average of this data set, equations based upon molecular volume should provide better estimates.

Fitzpatrick et al. (2004) reanalysed the same data set as that of Patel et al. (2002) and discussed variability in the database. In addition to problems associated with the K_p data themselves, they asserted that there may be problems in using partition coefficient values for ionizable compounds determined consistent with guidelines (e.g. OECD Test Guideline 117; OECD 2004d) that require pH adjustment to prevent ionization, which may require conditions that are outside the normal physiological range encountered in transdermal transport (see also O'Neill & Fitzpatrick, 2004). As long as permeation of the ionized species is much smaller than that of the non-ionized species, then permeation will be primarily by the non-ionized species (Vecchia & Bunge, 2003a). This topic of ionizable compounds is also discussed in chapter 4.

Details of all the recent QSPeR models are beyond the scope of this document. Table 8 gives an overview of some of the studies and the sources of data used. A more comprehensive listing is given in Vecchia & Bunge (2003a), which includes a comparison of several additional QSPeR models with data.

10.1.2.3 Other data sets

A few QSAR studies have been performed on smaller data sets that were not part of the Flynn (1990) data set. Several of these are based on congeneric series of compounds, typically drugs, and assess their permeation rates. As the emphasis of this document is on chemical risk assessment, these smaller studies are not described in detail here.

Several studies have investigated the percutaneous absorption of PAHs. That of van Rooij et al. (1995) was based on 10 PAHs. A more extensive study (Roy et al., 1998) included 60 PAHs, all of which were extremely hydrophobic (lowest K_{ow} being 4.00). A negative correlation was found between the percentage of applied dose that penetrated the rat skin in vitro after 24 h and hydrophobicity. The data were reanalysed by Gute et al. (1999), who modelled molecular weight alone rather than K_{ow} against percutaneous absorption of PAHs, probably because molecular weight and K_{ow} are highly correlated for these compounds.

10.1.3 Other approaches to QSPeR

Hostynek & Magee (1997) correlated human skin absorption data determined in vivo under different experimental conditions for a set of 28 diverse chemical compounds with experimental permeability coefficients obtained for 8 compounds in vitro on human skin and with permeability coefficients calculated according to a modified Potts–Guy algorithm. They suggested that both the vehicle in which the chemical is delivered and the degree of occlusion of the device were important. The most significant correlation was seen for a subset of 10 semi-occluded applications of different compounds.

10.1.4 Variability of data and its relevance for QSPeRs

Taking the values for estradiol reviewed by Johnson et al. (1995) — excluding that from Scheuplein et al. (1969), which has been questioned (Moss & Cronin, 2002; Moss et al., 2002) — there is a variability of about 25% in permeability coefficients, which, due to the inherent variability of the tissue and interlaboratory differences (and temperature differences), is tolerated by those working in the field. For deriving QSPeRs, however, such variance is detrimental, not just to the development of a robust and biologically relevant model, but also to its credibility and value in the question of predictability of skin permeability for other compounds (Moss et al., 2002). Permeability coefficients will differ from one solvent to another, depending upon the solubility of the penetrant and also the effect of the solvent on the skin. Nearly all of the published QSPeRs are for compounds in water, chiefly because these are the data that are available to model. As a result, the nature of drug–vehicle interactions and the choice of solvent are not considered by the existing QSPeRs (Walters & Brain, 2000). Strategies for making vehicle-to-vehicle adjustments have been proposed (e.g. USEPA, 1992), but more experimental studies supporting these methods are needed.

10.1.5 Statistical analysis (linear vs non-linear) methods

For many QSARs, including QSPeRs, regression analysis is the statistical method of choice, being simple, transparent, and highly portable (Cronin & Schultz, 2001). However, there are a number of disadvantages to using this method: in particular, firstly, the linear technique, and secondly, that it is adversely affected by collinearity between independent variables (e.g. log K_{ow} and molecular weight). It is not clear whether regression analysis is a suitable technique for the development of QSPeRs; nor is it clear whether linearity is appropriate for modelling of highly hydrophilic and hydrophobic molecules. Other possibilities would be partial least squares and artificial neural network modelling (Degim et al., 2003).

10.1.6 Selection of chemicals for further tests on dermal penetration

Ideally, for development of QSARs, the process of selection of chemicals should include a chemometric analysis to ensure that those compounds provide the maximum possible information. If the physicochemical descriptors for the QSPeR are restricted to log K_{ow}

and molecular weight, then selection of chemicals is easier than for a multivariant system. The current database must be critically analysed to decide how representative it is and what deficiencies it has (Jones et al., 2004). The European Chemical Industry Council (CEFIC) Working Group (and others before them) noted that there may not be a linear relationship between permeability coefficient and hydrophobicity for the complete range of log K_{ow} values. Polar compounds with low K_{ow} values may penetrate skin by pathways that are not represented by K_{ow}. At high K_{ow} values, the viable epidermis will restrict permeation. This is part of the rationale behind recommendations of EC (2004) that a reduced default absorption be assumed when log K_{ow} is either less than −1 or greater than 4. However, this recommendation does not account for the effect of K_{ow} on water solubility, and, as discussed in chapter 4, maximum flux (e.g. the product of K_p from water and the water solubility) may be a more suitable indicator for dermal absorption potential.

10.1.7 Applicability domain for QSPeR

The applicability domain for QSAR is defined as "the physicochemical, structural, or biological space, knowledge or information on which the training set of the model has been developed, and for which it is applicable to make predictions for new compounds" (Jaworska et al., 2003). At present, no formal methods exist to define such an applicability domain. However, it is accepted practice that a QSAR should not be used to make predictions outside of its applicability domain (Cronin & Schultz, 2001). If a global QSPeR can be based on log K_{ow} and molecular weight, then an applicability domain may be defined relatively easily and may be shown graphically on a two-dimensional plot of log K_{ow} and molecular weight, which will probably be elliptical in shape, due to the paucity of low molecular weight molecules that are hydrophobic. The CEFIC Working Group recommended that the applicability domain should be defined for any QSPeR developed and that all predictions should be made only for chemicals within the applicability domain (Jones et al., 2004).

10.1.8 Maximum fluxes

Maximum flux QSPeRs are of particular value, as they apply to all vehicles that do not affect the skin adversely. A prediction of fluxes less than the maximum flux can be made on the basis of concentrations being expressed in terms of fractional solubilities for a given vehicle (Roberts et al., 2002). Maximum flux QSARs are generally based on the premise that transport through the stratum corneum can be related to the solubility of solutes in the stratum corneum, the diffusivity of solutes through the stratum corneum, and the presence of any interfacial resistances (Kasting et al., 1987; Magnusson et al., 2004a). While the fuller expression of the QSAR with molecular weight and log K_{ow} is intrinsically non-linear, the resulting regression is only marginally better than a linear relationship between log of the maximum flux (mol/cm^2 per hour) and molecular weight ($P < 0.001$, $n = 278$, $r^2 = 0.688$) (Magnusson et al., 2004a):

$$\text{Log } J_{\text{max}} = 4.52 - 0.0141 \text{ MW} \quad \text{[Equation 10]}$$

10.1.9 *Rules as an alternative to QSPeRs*

QSARs can also be analysed using principal components analysis and related techniques. Such an approach has been used to broadly model skin permeability and cytotoxicity and to discriminate between corrosive and non-corrosive chemicals (Barratt, 1995a,b). Skin penetrants have also been classified as "good", "bad", or "intermediate", based on rules defined by the solutes' physicochemical properties (Magnusson et al., 2004b). Such rules are more commonly used to predict the likely skin toxicity of compounds (e.g. Gerner et al., 2004).

10.2 Mathematical modelling

Mechanistically based models relate dermal absorption to physicochemical parameters, such as diffusion coefficients and partition coefficients, that depend on the diffusing chemical and the vehicle. These parameters can be derived from experiments or estimated using QSAR equations developed from experimental measurements. In the simplest models, skin is treated as a single pseudo-homogeneous barrier, represented as either a membrane or a stirred compartment. More complex models include additional skin layers, such as the viable epidermis and/or dermis.

Membrane-based mathematical models have been developed for calculating the rate and extent of dermal absorption for a variety of exposure situations (Roberts & Anissimov, 2005). Cleek & Bunge (1993) described one- and two-membrane models for the skin that represent the stratum corneum alone and in combination with the viable epidermis. In these models, it was assumed that the chemical concentration in the vehicle remained constant during the exposure. Bunge and colleagues (Cleek & Bunge, 1993; Bunge & Cleek, 1995; Bunge et al., 1995; Bunge & McDougal, 1999) also proposed strategies for estimating the physicochemical parameters that these models require when the vehicle is water. These models were included in documents by the USEPA (1992, 2004b). Reddy et al. (1998) extended these models to include the loss of chemical in the skin at the end of exposure by desquamation of the stratum corneum. In this model, they included the barrier effect of the viable epidermis and again assumed that the chemical concentration did not change during the exposure. This desquamation is likely to affect the stratum corneum reservoir effect for only the most lipophilic solutes (Roberts et al., 2004).

The penetration of a volatile compound or mixture from the skin surface after topical application involves both diffusion in the stratum corneum and evaporation from the vehicle. Kasting's group (Kasting & Saiyasombati, 2001; Saiyasombati & Kasting, 2003; Kasting & Miller, 2006) have described this process and developed appropriate models. Stempfer & Bunge (2004) have also presented a one-membrane model of the stratum corneum, allowing for evaporation of absorbed chemical. They showed that for volatile compounds, a significant fraction of the chemical in the stratum corneum at the end of the exposure will probably evaporate. For semi-volatile compounds, the amount that would evaporate will depend on both the vapour pressure (which affects evaporation rate) and the absorption rate through the skin.

In the Skinperm model for prediction of the permeation of substances (Skinperm 3.1 model; Wilschut et al., 1995; ten Berge, 2005), the skin was considered to consist of the following compartments: protein layer of the stratum corneum, lipid layer of the stratum corneum, and aqueous layer below the stratum corneum. The overall permeation coefficients were expressed mathematically as a complex of permeation coefficients, representing the permeation through these layers. The regression coefficients were derived from the experimental results and were based on the database established by Wilschut and co-workers. The values of the regression coefficients in the model were: b1 = −1.736; b2 = 0.7219; b3 = −0.059 93; b4 = 0.000 297 6; and b5 = 4.209. For the permeation coefficient, the 95% confidence limits were provided. These 95% confidence limits were based on the original variances and covariances of the derived regression equation of the QSAR predicting the permeation coefficient, dependent on the octanol/water partition coefficient and on the molecular weight. The model predicts, among other parameters, the cumulative amount absorbed into the skin (ABS_{skin}) and K_p. In order to calculate the time-weighted average skin flux ($J_{skin,\ average,\ model}$), the value of ABS_{skin} is divided by the exposure concentration, C_{exp}, the exposure duration, $t_{exp,\ der}$, and the exposed skin area, A_{skin}. An example of the use of this model with xylene is given in Kezic et al. (2004).

The recent modelling efforts by Krüse & Kezic (2004) allow for variation of concentration in an aqueous vehicle and include barrier contributions from both the stratum corneum and viable epidermis. Like Bunge and colleagues, Krüse & Kezic (2004) have assumed local equilibrium at the water–stratum corneum and stratum corneum–viable epidermis interfaces, described by partition coefficients and diffusion coefficients in each layer. The model is based on Fick's law of diffusion within each layer (and based on a diffusion coefficient for the chemical in each layer). The model has more parameters (to be fitted), but it describes the time course of permeation more thoroughly, and it is in principle more appropriate for predicting the consequences of non-steady-state doses. It has been fitted to data describing the time course of permeation of chemical into the skin in vitro.

The rate-limiting step of permeation is often diffusion through the stratum corneum. However, for some compounds (highly lipophilic compounds) that have a much higher solubility in the skin than in water (e.g. by a factor of 1000), the diffusion within the aqueous solution towards the skin surface may become a rate-limiting factor (Kasting & Robinson, 1993).

Mathematical modelling plays a key role in linking the permeability coefficient obtained from tests under idealized, infinite dose conditions (i.e. steady-state conditions) to those that will occur under the finite dose conditions more typical of occupational exposure (i.e. non-steady-state conditions).

Mathematical modelling has also been used to estimate dermal absorption of contaminants from, for example, water and soil. USEPA (1992) presents a two-compartment diffusion model for estimating dermal absorption of contaminants from water. USEPA (2004b) presents a modification to this model that accounts for losses of lipophilic compounds, which are absorbed in the stratum corneum and lost via desquamation.

Mathematical models have also been described for predicting dermal absorption from chemicals. USEPA (2004b) presents the traditional per cent absorbed approach for estimating dermal absorption from soils. More mechanistic models are described in Bunge & Parks (1998).

10.3 Mathematical pharmacokinetic models of percutaneous penetration

Recent reviews on mathematical pharmacokinetic models of percutaneous penetration are given by Roberts et al. (1999), McCarley & Bunge (1998a,b, 2001), Reddy et al. (1998), and Roberts & Anissimov (2005). The rate constants in compartmental pharmacokinetic models can be related to the physicochemical parameters, such as diffusion coefficients and partition coefficients of the stratum corneum and additional skin layers. However, especially in a one-compartmental representation of the skin, these relationships require simplifying assumptions, which are sometimes not fully stated. McCarley & Bunge (1998a,b, 2000, 2001) and Reddy et al. (1998) have derived several different pharmacokinetic rate constants based on different assumptions applied in compartmental models. They have also showed that calculations made with these different rate constants can sometimes produce significantly different results that are not consistent with membrane models of skin, which the compartmental pharmacokinetic models are meant to simulate. Reddy et al. (1998) have presented model calculations that include concentration variation in the vehicle and blood when the stratum corneum is the rate-limiting barrier. Additional calculations made by Roberts et al. (1999) have validated and extended this analysis.

In such models, the algebraic equations that accurately represent the partition processes and diffusion migration of a molecule through the different layers of the stratum corneum are written down and solved within certain chosen simplifying assumptions (Fitzpatrick et al., 2004). Such a set of equations has been solved analytically for both steady-state and non-steady-state transport through a two-membrane composite representing the lipophilic stratum corneum and the hydrophilic viable epidermis layers (Cleek & Bunge, 1993). Recently, Wang et al. (2006) have described a two-dimensional microscopic model of the stratum corneum, recognizing varying hydration and permeability of corneocytes. A key outcome of the model is a mechanistic description of the dependency of the stratum corneum permeability coefficient on the octanol/water partition coefficient and other parameters.

Estimates of dermal absorption are used in exposure assessment to calculate the internal dose of persons contacting, for example, pesticides and are a critical part of risk assessments. An exponential saturation model with a lag time was validated against a classic dermal absorption study of 12 pesticides administered to human volunteers. The model gave dermal absorption estimates consistent with reported values in the literature (Thongsinthusak et al., 1999).

In occupational exposure to toxic chemicals, dermal absorption may result from multiple short-term exposures as well as from long-term exposures. Corish et al. (2004) describe the application of two diffusion-type numerical models of percutaneous penetration to non-steady-state time course data generated by participants in the EDETOX project. The first is a new numerical model developed by J. Krüse (Krüse & Kezic, 2004) and implemented using the Berkeley Madonna package (http://www.berkeleymadonna.com). The second is an implementation using Mathematica (http://www.wolfram.com) of an existing pair of models developed by Anissimov & Roberts (1999, 2000, 2001) (see also Roberts et al., 1999; Roberts & Anissimov, 2005). Both models allow finite and infinite doses to be modelled.

11. USE OF DERMAL PENETRATION STUDIES IN RISK ASSESSMENT

Risk assessment is a process by which the extent of exposure is compared against the hazard (intrinsic toxicity) of the chemical to determine whether it is likely to result in harm to the exposed individual(s). Exposure to a chemical can be by oral, inhalational, or dermal routes; however, in an occupational and many environmental and consumer settings, the latter two are the major routes.

To determine the hazard or intrinsic toxicity of a chemical, a comprehensive array of toxicity tests is performed, from which the critical effect and a "no-observed-adverse-effect level" (NOAEL) are derived. An uncertainty factor (sometimes called a safety factor), which is chosen in recognition of intra- and interspecies variability (maximum 10-fold for each) and the adequacy of the toxicological database (IPCS, 1994), is applied to the NOAEL, to give a guidance value. Alternatively, a margin of safety of exposure can be calculated for a specific scenario by comparing the NOAEL with the actual exposure conditions.

Since most laboratory animal testing is by oral administration, but the predominant route of exposure for pesticides, for example, is by skin absorption, the extent of dermal absorption needs to be determined to perform an occupational risk assessment (route-to-route extrapolation).

Although the scope of this document is focused on dermal absorption assuming normal healthy skin, it should be recognized that both the intrinsic local toxicity of the chemical and the skin condition can influence the degree to which the chemical is absorbed (see chapters 3 and 12).

Skin irritation, sensitization, and phototoxicity are part of the formal risk assessment process for local skin effects. These effects most commonly occur after acute or short-term exposure. Personal protective equipment (e.g. gloves/coveralls) is recommended when appropriate.

Assessment of dermal absorption is an important aspect of the overall risk assessment of chemicals coming in contact with the skin. One reason is that inhalation exposures to chemicals have decreased as a result of improved control technologies and reduction of occupational exposure limits (OELs), thereby increasing the contribution of dermal exposure. In certain scenarios, dermal exposure may be greater than respiratory exposure, and intoxications due to skin exposure have been documented. The skin is not an almost impermeable barrier to chemicals, as was originally thought. Now there are many databases describing skin permeation of chemicals (see chapter 9). Determination of dermal absorption is a key element of the risk assessment of pesticides, biocides, cosmetics, pharmaceuticals, and industrial chemicals. The potential exposure can occur during the manufacturing process, transport, and the end use of products. In addition, exposure to chemicals can occur in the environment.

For pesticides, biocides, cosmetics, and industrial chemicals, the internal exposure is calculated on the basis of relative absorption (percentage of dose applied) under realistic exposure conditions (e.g. area dose and formulation). Although conventional risk assessments are usually not performed for pharmaceuticals because of the benefit derived through deliberate dosing, the exposure can be calculated using plasma AUC, excretion data, and pharmacological effect data. The peak exposure is defined by the maximum plasma concentration, whereas total exposure is defined by the AUC. Other methods of calculation of internal dose include steady-state flux estimations and biologically based modelling (McDougal & Boeniger, 2002). At present, these methods are not widely applied in risk assessment, with the exception of dermal exposure to large amounts of chemicals — e.g. incidents at work and contaminated (swimming) water (Walker et al., 1996; Moody, 1998).

11.1 Decision-making process for setting dermal absorption values

There are various ways to determine the actual skin absorption of a substance, and the methodology for this has been described in previous chapters (in vitro experimentation, in vivo animal studies, and studies with human volunteers). In addition, order-of-magnitude estimates of dermal absorption can be made by considering data on physicochemical properties of the substance, such as molecular weight and log K_{ow} (chapter 10). The use of these data in risk assessment may vary depending on the chemical or product area, and guidance has been developed by various regulatory agencies. This section provides an overview of the current practices.

11.1.1 Default values

In the absence of any experimental dermal absorption data, one should assume the worst-case scenario, in which 100% of the chemical at a relevant dose will be absorbed. If this initial, very conservative, risk assessment indicates that the exposure level is acceptable/tolerable, a quantitive estimate of dermal absorption is not required. Otherwise, an assessment of dermal absorption is the next step.

In Europe, regulatory authorities involved in risk assessment are using a rule based on molecular weight and log K_{ow} to distinguish between chemicals with high and low potential for dermal absorption (EC, 2003, 2004):

- 10% dermal absorption for those chemicals with a molecular weight > 500 *and* log K_{ow} smaller than −1 or higher than 4;
- otherwise assume 100% dermal absorption.

The reason for assuming 10% as the lower limit was that the data presented in the literature indicated the occurrence of dermal absorption for tested compounds even beyond the extremes of log K_{ow} and/or molecular weight values (EC, 2003, 2004). However, by expert judgement, a deviation from these 10% or 100% values can be chosen on a case-by-case basis, taking into account all the data available (e.g. water solubility, ionogenic state, molecular volume, oral absorption, and dermal area dose in exposure situations in practice). Appropriate values for oral absorption can be obtained by absorption, distribution, metabolism, and excretion (ADME) studies, using low dose levels.

[*Comment of the IPCS Task Group*: The validity of using the physicochemical properties to obtain the default criteria is unclear. A preferable method may be to use dermal absorption rates based on the QSAR between maximum flux and molecular weight or rules for good, bad, and intermediate permeants (see chapters 4 and 10). It is recognized that this rate will usually be an overestimate of dermal absorption, as maximum flux does not take into account lag time and relevant dosing conditions.]

In Europe, results from acute toxicity studies (dermal and oral) are not considered suitable for estimation of skin absorption (EC, 2004). Acute doses, especially those using gavage administration, result in relatively fast oral absorption, resulting in a peak concentration in the body, whereas absorption after dermal exposure is generally more gradual. Differences in toxicity between oral and dermal exposure could be the result of different "first-pass" effects in the liver and the skin. The North American Free Trade Agreement Technical Working Group on Pesticides agreed that in the absence of an acceptable in vivo dermal absorption study, dermal absorption and absorption via the oral route would be considered equivalent (i.e. up to 100%) (Hakkert et al., 2005). The California Department of Pesticide Regulation uses a default of 50% for regulatory purposes based on an upper-bound estimate of dermal absorption of 40 pesticides, which were obtained from studies in rats (Donahue, 1996).

For the occupational risk assessment of pesticides in Australia, a default dermal absorption value of 100% is usually used in the absence of any chemical-specific experimental data. However, this value may be reduced if there are suitable dermal absorption data from a related chemical (i.e. same class). Other factors include a consideration of the molecular size or a comparison of oral and dermal repeated-dose toxicity of the substance (APVMA, 1997).

11.1.2 Measured values

The most reliable data for determining absorption through human skin are obtained from in vivo human volunteer studies performed under occupationally relevant test conditions (Ross et al., 2005). These could be both controlled volunteer studies and biomonitoring studies. In addition, some cosmetic ingredients have been studied under controlled in-use conditions (e.g. Nohynek et al., 2006). For technical and ethical reasons, the conduct of these studies is limited and closely regulated.

Recently, OECD test guidelines for in vivo (OECD Test Guideline 427) and in vitro (OECD Test Guideline 428) dermal absorption studies have been adopted (OECD, 2004b,c) to encourage a harmonized approach in their conduct. In addition, criteria on the performance of in vitro studies have been developed in the cosmetics area (SCCNFP, 2003b). In all guidelines, it is emphasized that it is essential that studies reflect the anticipated exposure situation (e.g. dose, formulation, exposure time). It should be realized that the data on external exposure are often measured or estimated averages over the total exposed area. Since skin absorption is dependent on the applied dose, improved accuracy of exposure data will lead to more realistic skin absorption data.

In animal studies, absorption is determined on the basis of the excretion profiles and the amount in the carcass of the laboratory animal at the end of the experiment (see chapter 7). The skin-bound dose is critical for the calculation of the dermal absorption in in vivo studies (Chu et al., 1996; EC, 2004). The decision about the quantity that remains bound in the skin can be based on the excretion curve — a decline of radioactivity in the excreta at the end of the experiment indicates that the dose at the application site may not become completely systemically available (Thongsinthusak et al., 1999; see chapters 7 and 12).

In vitro dermal absorption studies on pesticides have been used for risk assessment purposes for more than 20 years within the EU under Directive 91/414. Other regulatory authorities are increasingly accepting in vitro data as part of the risk assessment process. Despite the fact that in vitro studies have been shown to be in generally good agreement with in vivo dermal absorption (chapter 8), there is still controversy over how in vitro data are used in risk assessment. An important issue of concern is the presence of (lipophilic) test substances remaining in the skin at the end of the experiment. Provided that skin levels are included as absorbed, results from in vitro methods are considered adequate for risk assessment (in the absence of in vivo data). However, the fate of the compound remaining in the skin is important and may need be to be determined in additional measurements (see section 6.4 and chapter 12).

In vitro dermal absorption studies are preferably carried out with human skin preparations; pig skin is considered a suitable alternative. In vitro studies with rat skin can be used, but this leads to a more conservative estimate, as absorption by human skin is usually lower than that by rat skin (EC, 2004). If appropriate dermal absorption data are available from rats in vivo and for rat and human skin in vitro, the in vivo human absorption value can be calculated according to the following equation (EC, 2004; van Ravenzwaay & Leibold, 2004):

$$\text{In vivo human absorption} = \frac{\text{in vivo rat absorption} \times \text{in vitro human absorption}}{\text{in vitro rat absorption}}$$

11.1.3 Values from mathematical skin permeation models (e.g. QSARs/QSPeRs)

As the present QSARs are based on absorption data from chemicals in aqueous solutions at infinite dose, it is important that methods are developed to apply the data to realistic exposure scenarios (low dose, formulated substances, repeated exposure, mixtures with potential cumulative or synergistic effects). The use of QSARs may prove to be a useful screening tool and may prove valuable for a group of closely related pure substances (EC, 2003; Jones et al., 2004) for predicting dermal absorption potential (see chapter 10).

11.2 Use of relative absorption values versus flux (and their derived permeability coefficients)

Dermal absorption of chemicals is most often expressed as a percentage of the dose that is in contact with the skin. Until now, fluxes (and the derived permeability coefficient values) have not been incorporated in occupational risk assessment in the United States, but are used to estimate the degree of an acute exposure from a large amount/volume of a chemical (incidental splash, contaminated swimming water) (Walker et al., 1996). However, the USEPA is promulgating a final rule under the Toxic Substances Control Act (TSCA) that requires manufacturers, importers, and processors of 34 chemicals to conduct in vitro dermal absorption rate studies. These chemicals are of interest to the Occupational Safety and Health Administration of the United States Department of Labour, and the data will be used to evaluate the need for skin designations for these chemicals (USEPA, 2004a).

Methods for conducting dermal risk assessments for the water and soil pathways at Superfund sites are given in USEPA (2004b). The document gives K_p values for over 200 organic chemical contaminants in water, calculated using a mathematical model based on absorption data from Flynn's (1990) data set on 90 hydrophilic chemicals (see chapter 10). For guidance on permeability coefficients for inorganic compounds, USEPA (2004b) presents a table compiled from specific chemical experimental data as modified from USEPA (1992) and Hostynek et al. (1998). The USEPA (2004b) guidance document presents recommended default exposure values for all variables for the dermal–water and dermal–soil pathways for Superfund sites. The modelling of dermal absorption from soils and powders in vivo has recently been reviewed (Bunge et al., 2005).

An approach for deciding whether to consider dermal absorption in a risk assessment is by comparing it with other pathways of exposure. For example, for a contaminated drinking-water scenario, the dermal pathway (i.e. bathing) is evaluated only if the screening analysis suggests that it will contribute at least 10% of the dose from drinking the water (USEPA, 2004b).

11.3 Other topics related to risk assessment

Harmonization of skin notation and dermal absorption in susceptible populations are discussed in chapter 12 on controversial topics.

12. CONTROVERSIAL TOPICS IN THE ASSESSMENT OF DERMAL ABSORPTION

Although there has been a movement towards harmonization of methodology (OECD, 2004a,b,c), there are still many topics in dermal absorption assessment that are controversial. This chapter touches on some of these issues and refers the reader, where necessary, to the relevant sections in the present document or to other sources of information.

12.1 QSARs/QSPeRs

The OECD guidelines are not strict protocols. However, the acceptance and use of these guidelines should lead to a more reliable database. Can reliable QSPeRs be constructed from such an improved database, or are stricter protocols necessary (e.g. that suggested by a CEFIC Working Group; Jones et al., 2004) (see chapter 10 and Appendix 2)?

The acceptance of QSARs/QSPeRs themselves is still a matter of controversy. On the one hand, dermal absorption data are lacking for thousands of chemicals; on the other hand, variability of data is controversial. Further, guidance is needed on how to use QSAR data in risk assessment. At present, most QSARs give estimates of K_p values (or relative absorption over 24 h), which need to be "translated" into a parameter that can be applied in risk assessment.

12.2 Reduction of intralaboratory/interlaboratory variation

There is still a debate going on about how in vitro data could or should be used in risk assessment. An evaluation of available data on in vitro dermal absorption was performed under the auspices of the OECD (2000). Because the available studies comparing the in vitro and in vivo test results contained many variables (different species, thickness and types of skin, exposure duration, vehicles, etc.), an evaluation/consensus was found to be difficult. Some of the variables in in vitro determinations and in in vivo experiments were discussed in chapter 6 and chapter 7, respectively. Studies on inter- and intralaboratory variation (chapter 8) reinforce the need to conduct carefully controlled in vitro and in vivo dermal absorption studies. Some of these topics (e.g. skin thickness, vehicle effects, appropriate receptor fluids, tape stripping) have also been addressed in a recent European project (i.e. EDETOX; see section A2.3 in Appendix 2).

In general, studies have shown that properly conducted in vitro measurements can be used to predict in vivo absorption (chapter 8). The acceptance of in vitro measurements in lieu of in vivo studies by regulatory authorities (chapter 11) necessitates controlled study conditions using accepted protocols.

12.3 Consequences of reservoir effect for risk assessment

Another controversial issue is the presence of test substance in the various skin layers — i.e. absorbed into the skin but not passed into the receptor fluid (see sections 3.5 and 6.4). In particular, very lipophilic compounds are difficult to investigate in vitro due to their low solubility in most receptor fluids. If the amount retained in the skin is also counted as being absorbed, a more acceptable but conservative estimate can be made. Water-soluble substances can be tested more accurately in vitro because they more readily diffuse into the receptor fluid. If skin levels are included in the overall per cent absorption figure, results from in vitro methods seem to adequately reflect those from in vivo experiments and support their use as a replacement of in vivo testing (EC, 2003).

Different approaches are taken by different bodies. ECETOC (1993) base their measurements of percutaneous absorption on receptor fluids only. In the cosmetic guidelines issued by the European Cosmetic Toiletry and Perfumery Association (COLIPA) (Diembeck et al., 1999) and the SCCNFP (2003b), the material remaining in the epidermis and dermis, in addition to that in the receptor fluid, is considered as being systemically available, but not the test substance remaining in the stratum corneum at the end of the study. In OECD Test Guideline 428 (OECD, 2004c), skin absorption may sometimes be expressed using receptor fluid data alone. However, when the test substance remains in the skin at the end of the study (e.g. lipophilic test substances), it may need to be included in the total amount absorbed. The OECD (2004a) guidance document notes that skin fractionation (e.g. by tape stripping) may be performed to further define the localization of the test substances within the skin as required by the objectives of the study. Alternatively, distribution within the skin can be determined by taking vertical sections and using autoradiography or other analytical techniques to visualize the test substance.

A recent publication has discussed this topic and concludes that when the movement of chemicals from a skin reservoir to the receptor fluid is shown to occur, it is appropriate to add skin levels to receptor fluid values to obtain a more realistic estimate of dermal absorption (Yourick et al., 2004).

12.4 Relevance of percutaneous measurements to data required by risk assessors: finite and infinite exposures

Ideally, estimates of dermal absorption required by risk assessors should be as close as possible to real exposure conditions. To achieve this, experiments should be conducted under finite dose conditions, using vehicles, concentrations of chemicals, and periods of exposure that reflect in-use conditions (Benford et al., 1999; EC, 2004). In practice, most in vitro dermal absorption studies are carried out under infinite exposure conditions. At present, there are attempts to use modelling to link permeability coefficients measured under infinite exposure (steady-state) conditions to conditions more typical of occupational exposure (non-steady-state conditions) (see also chapter 10; section A2.3.4 in Appendix 2; Jones et al., 2004; Krüse & Kezic, 2004).

12.5 Single- versus multiple-exposure regimes

It is suggested that experiments using multiple-dosing regimes would be more comparable with occupational exposure scenarios. However, most data from dermal absorption studies are from single-exposure regimes. Data on the effects of repeated exposure are scarce and conflicting. Some data show that repeated exposures may alter dermal absorption (e.g. Roberts & Horlock, 1978; Wester & Maibach, 1996). However, others show no differences. For example, the effects of single and multiple dosing (for 14–21 days) on the dermal absorption of six test compounds (methylprednisolone aceponate, azone, malathion, estradiol, hydrocortisone, and testosterone) have been compared. No significant changes in absorption were observed following multiple dosing (Wester et al., 1983, 1994; Bucks et al., 1985; Tauber & Matthes, 1992). Pendlington et al. (2004) found that in a repeated-dose experiment with caffeine, the amount recovered from each skin compartment mirrored the number of doses applied.

12.6 Barrier integrity test for skin barrier function of human skin in skin penetration tests

OECD Test Guideline 428 (OECD, 2004c) recommends the use of a barrier integrity test when performing skin penetration studies for regulatory submission. There is much debate at the moment as to whether barrier integrity tests actually correlate to epidermal properties (Gordon Research Conference, 2005). If skin samples do not exhibit a permeability coefficient K_p for tritiated water above 2.5×10^{-3} cm/h, they are rejected as being "damaged". In a recent study (Roper et al., 2004) on K_p values from 1110 human skin samples, 230 (21%) were rejected because they did not fulfil the barrier integrity criteria. However, it is likely that many of these rejected samples were atypical rather than damaged, resulting in an underestimation of absorption in such an individual. Further, this is an unnecessary wastage of valuable human skin samples, leading to a truncation of the actual population frequency distribution of K_p at high K_p (see also section 6.2).

12.7 Dermal absorption in susceptible populations

Risk assessment of dermal exposure is mostly related to healthy, adult individuals. However, skin contact with chemicals occurs in everyday life, and all parts of a population are potentially exposed.

Concern for children as a potentially susceptible population for exposure to toxic environmental agents has increased dramatically in the last few years (Daston et al., 2004). As full-term neonates have a well developed stratum corneum, it is generally believed that the age of the child has little bearing on dermal permeability (USEPA, 1992). However, the stratum corneum of premature infants is less effective than that of full-term infants or adults (Barker et al., 1987; USEPA, 1992), and dermal absorption has to be considered in scenarios where these neonates are dermally exposed to contaminants present in bath water or to chemicals in hygienic or diaper rash products. Furthermore, risks from dermal exposure to environmental chemicals may differ between children and adults for a variety of reasons, including differing behavioural patterns, anatomical and physiological differences, and developmental differences of vital organs such as the brain, which may result in different end organ effects (Mancini, 2005).

Enhanced dermal absorption has also been reported in skin affected by disease. Certain genetic defects in lipid metabolism or in the protein components of the stratum corneum produce scaly or ichthyotic skin with abnormal barrier lipid structure and function (Madison, 2003). The inflammatory skin diseases psoriasis and atopic dermatitis also show decreased barrier function. The psoriatic skin allows more penetration of not only low molecular weight substances but also large proteins (Schaefer et al., 1977; Gould et al., 2003). In atopic dermatitis epidermis, a significant decrease in the ceramide content correlates with an increased rate of water loss at the skin surface — a sign of an impaired barrier (Humbert, 2003). This is consistent with the findings of Jakasa et al. (2005), who found increased stratum corneum penetration of polyethylene glycols of a wide range of molecular weights through the clinically normal skin of atopic dermatitis patients. Abnormal barrier functions of clinically normal skin in atopic dermatitis were also reported by Hata et al. (2002), who found increased dermal absorption of hydrophilic dyes in the skin of atopic dermatitis patients. As a consequence, the impaired barrier functions of clinically normal skin in atopic dermatitis may predispose inflammatory processes evoked by irritants and allergens. This is a point of concern, since the prevalence of atopic dermatitis in industrialized countries is dramatically increasing.

Besides already damaged skin in disease, the skin barrier can be compromised in a wide variety of ways: physical damage (e.g. burned, shaved skin), chemical damage (e.g. detergents, solvents), occluded skin (e.g. wearing of gloves), increased hydration (e.g. excessive hand washing), and even psychological stress (USEPA, 1992; Choi et al., 2005). It has been shown that even slight damage to the skin achieved by sodium lauryl sulfate may lead to increased percutaneous penetration of chemicals covering a wide range of solubilities (Nielsen, 2005). Higher dermal absorption was also reported in skin damaged by acetone (Benfeldt et al., 1999; Tsai et al., 2001) and by tape stripping (Benfeldt et al., 1999; Tsai et al., 2003).

In conclusion, there is a line of evidence suggesting that the compromised skin barrier is not uncommon. This condition may make the skin more susceptible to irritants, sensitizers, and disease. In addition, a compromised barrier makes the skin more permeable and facilitates dermal uptake. Therefore, when evaluating the health risk associated with skin exposure, susceptible subgroups in the population should be taken into account. Furthermore, evaluation of potentially increased penetration due to chemical or physical damage should be included in risk assessment.

12.8 Skin notation

The skin notation was introduced almost 50 years ago as a qualitative indicator of hazard related to dermal absorption at work. It is designated if:

- skin exposure to a defined area, duration, etc. increases the systemic dose by a given percentage, compared with inhalation exposure at the OEL; and/or
- realistic dermal exposure at the workplace has been shown to cause adverse effects (Johanson, 2003).

A major complication is that the skin notation is often used as an instrument for risk management (Nielsen & Grandjean, 2004). Workplace exposure needs to be assessed in quantitative terms, and a qualitative hazard indicator, such as the skin notation, is not very useful for risk assessment or risk management. It has been suggested that skin notation should relate to the potential for toxicity following relevant dermal exposure (Sartorelli, 2002; Nielsen & Grandjean, 2004).

In many countries, compounds considered a skin hazard are identified by skin notation on the list of OELs. In general, the notation has the purpose of drawing attention to the fact that cutaneous exposure to these compounds can significantly contribute to total systemic exposure. Irritating and corrosive compounds do not have a skin notation.

12.8.1 Skin notation criteria in different countries

Vague criteria and lack of good data have led to different classifications for the same chemical by different authorities and organizations. The criteria used to assign such skin notations vary considerably between countries and institutions and are generally qualitative (Johanson, 2005). The different criteria are shown in Table 9.

Table 9. Criteria for assigning a skin notation in different countries[a]

Country	Criteria used to assign a skin notation by that country
Denmark	"When known that the substance can be absorbed via skin"
Norway	"Substances that can be taken up via skin"
Finland	"Absorbed amounts and health risks cannot be evaluated only from air concentrations"
Sweden	"Substances easily taken up by the body via skin"
Germany (MAK)	"When dermal exposure increases the body burden"
EU (SCOEL)	"Substantial contribution to total body burden via dermal exposure"
USA (ACGIH)	"Potential significant contribution to overall exposure by the cutaneous route, including mucous membranes and the eyes, either by contact with vapours or, of probable greater significance, by direct skin contact with the substance"
The Netherlands (DECOS)	"More than 10% contribution to total exposure..."
European industry (ECETOC)	"More than 10% contribution to total exposure..."

ACGIH, American Conference of Governmental Industrial Hygienists; DECOS, Dutch Expert Committee on Occupational Standards; ECETOC, European Centre for Ecotoxicology & Toxicology of Chemicals; MAK, German Senate Commission on the Investigation of Health Hazards of Chemical Compounds in the Work Area; SCOEL, Scientific Committee for Occupational Exposure Limits.

[a] From Johanson (2003).

A review of the use of the skin notation employed by many of the world's health and safety authorities identified inconsistencies (Fiserova-Bergerova et al., 1990). For example, the United Kingdom Health and Safety Executive currently assigns a skin notation to over 120 chemicals, while the American Conference of Governmental Industrial Hygienists (ACGIH) applies the skin notation to over 160 substances (Semple, 2004). The ACGIH notations have been criticized in the past for inconsistencies in documentation. Varying criteria for assignment are due to a lack of information on dermal absorption rates of chemicals (Semple, 2004). The German criteria for designation of a skin notation (discussed by Drexler, 1998) are that the maximal allowable concentration (MAK) for the substance is not sufficient to protect dermally exposed persons from adverse effects on their health. The German definition has therefore introduced adverse health effects as part of the criterion, but does not include quantitative terms (Nielsen & Grandjean, 2004).

12.8.2 Quantitative approaches

Although the concept of comparing dermal uptake with uptake following inhalation is central to most skin notation definitions, the exact terminology has yet to be decided. One approach for a quantitative term is to consider the dermal LD_{50}. Chemicals with dermal LD_{50} values below 2000 mg/kg body weight are normally regarded as a health risk to humans (Nielsen & Grandjean, 2004). The present use of skin notation does not reflect this proposal, as only a few countries have included all such chemicals on their lists of chemicals with a skin notation. An inherent problem with LD_{50} values is that they refer only to acute toxicity, with death as the single registered outcome. Thus, an acute LD_{50} value will not cover non-lethal or chronic toxicity, accumulation, or the effects of repeated dosing (Nielsen & Grandjean, 2004). Fiserova-Bergerova et al. (1990) recommended two reference values as criteria for skin notation: 1) the dermal absorption potential, which relates to dermal absorption raising the dose of non-volatile or biological levels of volatile chemicals 30% above those observed during inhalation exposure to the threshold limit value / time-weighted average (TLV-TWA) only, and 2) the dermal toxicity potential, which triples biological levels as compared with levels observed during inhalation exposure to the TLV-TWA only. The Netherlands uses the criterion that dermal exposure of the hands and forearms for 1 h must lead to uptake exceeding 10% of that received by inhalation for 8 h at the OEL for a skin notation (Semple, 2004).

12.8.3 New approaches

A comparison of dermal absorption rates between OEL listed chemicals with skin notation showed variation by several orders of magnitude, and the contribution of dermal absorption ranged from negligible to a major fraction of the absorbed dose (Johanson, 2003). The current qualitative skin notation does not reflect this.

A dermal uptake index (D in Equation 11, pD in Equation 12) that relates the contributions of dermal absorption rate (P_{skin}) to the respiratory uptake rate via inhalation at the OEL (P_{resp}) has been proposed (Johanson, 2005):

$$D = (P_{skin}/P_{resp}) \cdot k \qquad \text{[Equation 11]}$$

$$pD = \log_{10}D + 8 \text{ (with 8 including the constant } k \text{ in Equation 11)} \qquad \text{[Equation 12]}$$

Dermal occupational exposure limits (DOELs) have also been proposed (Bos et al., 1998), in which a limit is related to the total dose deposited on the skin during a work shift (Semple, 2004). The uncertainties that may restrict the use of DOELs in quantitative risk assessment include:

- difficulty in evaluating the extent of contaminated skin;
- regional variations in skin permeability;
- lack of percutaneous penetration data; and
- influence of workers' behaviour on skin contamination (Sartorelli, 2002).

The National Institute for Occupational Safety and Health in the United States is currently revising its criteria for skin notation (S. Soderholm, personal communication, 2005). There is an obvious need for harmonization of the skin notation both within the EU and with the United States and a strong argument for a quantitative component.

12.9 Dermal absorption of nanoparticles

Nanoscale materials have at least one dimension less than 100 nm, a scale 1000 times smaller than most microscale materials tested to date. This significant reduction in size has resulted in topical products containing nanoscale materials and has generated concern about the potential nanoparticle skin exposure. Cosmetic products containing non-ghosting sunscreens and nano-liposome-based skin care products, certain window sprays, paints, varnishes, and coatings are examples of nanoscale products (SCENIHR, 2005). It is, however, unclear exactly how well nanoparticles will penetrate the skin and what their toxicological impact will be (Tsuji et al., 2006). Kim et al. (2004) have shown that, when nanoparticles are administered in the dermis, they localize to regional lymph nodes, potentially via skin macrophages and Langerhans cells, raising potential concern for immunomodulation if nanoparticles penetrate the skin. Tsuji et al. (2006) suggest that potential sources of toxicity are skin or organ cytotoxicity, long-term toxicity subsequent to accumulation in skin and other organs, metabolism to toxic particles, and toxicity of photoactivated nanoparticles.

Titanium dioxide and zinc oxide nanoparticles have been included in sunscreens, as they scatter UV A but not visible light and therefore enable a transparent sunscreen. Several studies of micro-scale and nanoscale materials have identified titanium in the epidermis and dermis following application of titanium dioxide–containing sunscreens, whereas other studies found metal oxide or fluorescent polystyrene nanoparticles only in the hair follicles and skin furrows and no material below the surface of the stratum corneum (Tan et al., 1996; Lademann et al., 1999, 2001; Alvarez-Roman et al., 2004). Lansdown & Taylor (1997) suggested that microfine titanium dioxide penetrates the skin when applied in castor oil, but their studies used rabbits. Bennat & Muller-Goymann (2000) suggested that titanium dioxide penetrates human skin when applied as an oil in water emulsion, with penetration being greater in hairy skin.

Microparticles have been identified in the lymph nodes and dermis of individuals who walked barefoot in African rift valleys and developed elephantiasis of the feet and legs, suggesting that external force may be necessary for particle penetration to occur (Corachan et al., 1988; Blundell et al., 1989). This association of external pressure with particle translocation was extended by in vitro studies demonstrating translocation of fluorescent particles, 1 μm or smaller, into the epidermis of flexed human skin, as at the wrist (Tinkle et al., 2003).

The importance of the surface characteristics of nanoscale materials was reinforced by recent studies of transcutaneous vaccine delivery (Kohli & Alpar, 2004). Whereas negatively charged fluorescent particles of 50 and 500 nm permeated pig skin, neutral and positively charged particles did not. Surprisingly, negatively charged 100- and 200-nm fluorescent particles also did not penetrate. Additional research found that the total concentration of charge was critical. Zeta potential and crystallinity are critical parameters for successful penetration of nanoscale lipid vesicles and lipid solid particles into the skin (Souto et al., 2004).

Nanoscale materials also display novel chemical and physical properties, and the interaction of these materials with biological systems is uncertain. Several studies demonstrate that the epidermis can respond physiologically to particulate exposure. An in vivo study demonstrated the development of murine immune hypersensitivity following cutaneous application of beryllium oxide particulate, and an in vitro study confirmed single wall carbon nanotube induction of oxidative stress in a keratinocyte cell line (Shvedova et al., 2003).

Solid lipid nanoparticles have been used since the early 1990s in cosmetic products as an alternative system to emulsions, liposomes, and polymeric nanoparticles. Muller et al. (2002) reviewed this area. To date, emphasis appears to have been placed on measuring the skin absorption of drugs incorporated in the solid lipid nanoparticles rather the penetration of solid lipid nanoparticles per se (Santos et al., 2002; Borgia et al., 2005). Solid lipid nanoparticles can lead to macrophage cytotoxicity at high concentrations but, in general, appear to be safe, toxicologically acceptable carrier systems (Scholer at al., 2000).

In conclusion, nanoscale material science is an emerging field in which the benefits and adverse consequences of exposure and dermal absorption are not understood. If hairy animals are used, this may lead to an overestimation of dermal absorption after nanoparticle application, as most nanoparticle absorption appears to be via the follicles. Objective research will be critical over the next 5–10 years to promote responsible development that maximizes positive biological interaction and minimal adverse health effects. In the interim, public and corporate concern for the environmental and human health and safety of nanomaterials and products is high. Assessment of exposure risk and dermal absorption requires careful evaluation of the composition of the nanomaterials, their physical and chemical properties, the potential for exposure, the magnitude of exposure, the conditions of exposure, and, if absorption proves to be significant, the route of exposure. Established risk assessment methodologies can be used to build a framework to evaluate the current nanomaterials; however, this framework should be dynamic and revised as new safety data become available.

13. CONCLUSIONS AND RECOMMENDATIONS

1. Human skin in vitro and in vivo should be universally recognized as the gold standard in dermal absorption risk assessment.

2. In vitro and in vivo human experimental studies using standardized, well controlled methods are needed to appropriately assess human dermal absorption of chemicals, including formulated products, that come into contact with the skin.

3. Further efforts are needed to improve and harmonize methodology in order to minimize variability in in vitro dermal absorption measurements. Interlaboratory comparative studies should include appropriate internal and external quality controls, i.e.:
   - use of a validated analytical technique;
   - use of a standard membrane and test solution as an additional control;
   - cross-check using pure reference chemicals;
   - confirmation of barrier integrity;
   - consistent and appropriate skin preparation; and
   - other recommendations of the OECD test guidelines (OECD, 2004a,c).

4. There should be more research aimed at addressing the lack of repeated-dose dermal absorption experiments that simulate relevant exposure conditions.

5. In risk assessment, maximum flux, either measured or estimated from molecular weight, should be used in preference to K_p or percentages of the chemical absorbed. Adjustment should be made to account for non-saturating exposure.

6. Collection of more data on highly lipophilic chemicals under in-use conditions is needed to facilitate understand-

ing of the effect of various vehicles, receptor fluids, and mixtures on results obtained in dermal absorption studies.

7. There is a need for more in vivo and in vitro data on the dermal absorption of chemicals in damaged skin (e.g. mechanical damage, UV damage, skin irritants, sensitizers, and solvents) and in diseased skin to assist the risk assessment process.

8. Greater efforts should be made to correlate in vitro and in vivo data and to develop reliable prediction models.

9. The regression of the absorption time course will always give a more accurate estimate of dermal absorption parameters than the usual techniques and may be more valuable in finite dose estimation, in comparing different dose exposure scenarios, and in extrapolating to different occupational exposure situations.

10. Further efforts to evaluate QSARs for risk assessment purposes and to prepare guidance on their use are encouraged. However, the inherent limitations of QSARs to mimic a highly complex biological process must be recognized, and approaches being developed in the pharmaceuticals area to model drug–skin component interactions hold promise for the future.

11. Databases containing measured and well defined skin absorption data are a key first step in development of QSARs and for research to improve understanding of the dermal absorption process for chemicals. Such databases have been developed by industry, researchers, and government institutions and should be supported, maintained, and updated. Means of sharing data should be explored, recognizing that in some instances the data are proprietary.

12. Noting that different sectors (pesticides, industrial chemicals, cosmetics, pharmaceuticals, etc.) have long-established but different usages for some key terms (e.g. permeation, penetration, absorption, resorption, systemic absorption), it is important that terms are clearly defined in

scientific articles to aid interpretation. Similarly, care needs to be taken in making comparisons between studies.

13. It needs to be recognized that emerging technologies such as nanoparticles may have unanticipated toxicological consequences following contact with the skin.

14. Development and standardization of non-invasive and semi-invasive human in vivo methods, such as stratum corneum stripping, Fourier transform infrared, Raman, multiphoton, and confocal spectroscopy, and microdialysis, should be encouraged.

REFERENCES

Abraham MH & Martins F (2004) Human skin permeation and partition: general linear free-energy relationship analyses. J Pharm Sci, **93**(6): 1508–1522.

Abraham MH, Chadha HS & Mitchell RC (1995) The factors that influence skin penetration of solutes. J Pharm Pharmacol, **47**: 8–16.

Abraham MH, Chadha HS, Martins F, Mitchell RC, Bradbury MW & Gratton JA (1999) Hydrogen bonding part 46: a review of the correlation and prediction of transport properties by an LFER method: physicochemical properties, brain penetration and skin permeability. Pestic Sci, **55**: 78–88.

Ahmed AR (1979) Dermatology — Epitomes of progress; Langerhans cell — epidermal macrophage. West J Med, **130**(2): 162.

Alberti I, Kalia YN, Naik A, Bonny JD & Guy RH (2001) In vivo assessment of enhanced topical delivery of terbinafine to human stratum corneum. J Control Release, **71**(3): 319–327.

Alvarez-Roman R, Naik A, Kalia YN, Guy RH & Fessi H (2004) Skin penetration and distribution of polymeric nanoparticles. J Control Release, **99**(1): 53–62.

Anderson BD & Raykar PV (1989) Solute structure–permeability relationships in human stratum corneum. J Invest Dermatol, **93**(2): 280–286.

Anderson C, Andersson T & Boman A (1998) Cutaneous microdialysis for human in vivo dermal absorption studies. In: Roberts MS & Walters KA eds. Dermal absorption and toxicity assessment. New York, Marcel Dekker, pp 231–244 (Drugs and the Pharmaceutical Sciences Vol. 91).

Anissimov YG & Roberts MS (1999) Diffusion modeling of percutaneous absorption kinetics. 1. Effects of flow rate, receptor sampling rate, and viable epidermal resistance for a constant donor concentration. J Pharm Sci, **88**(11): 1201–1209.

Anissimov YG & Roberts MS (2000) Diffusion modeling of percutaneous absorption kinetics. 1. Effects of flow rate, receptor sampling rate, and viable epidermal resistance for a constant donor concentration [erratum]. J Pharm Sci, **89**(1): 144.

Anissimov YG & Roberts MS (2001) Diffusion modeling of percutaneous absorption kinetics. 2. Finite vehicle volume and solvent deposited solids. J Pharm Sci, **90**(4): 504–520.

APVMA (1997) Occupational health and safety. Part 6 of Agricultural Requirement Series. Kingston, ACT, Australian Pesticides and Veterinary Medicines Authority, National Registration Authority for Agricultural and Veterinary Chemicals (http://www.apvma.gov.au/MORAG_ag/vol_3/part_6_OHS.pdf).

Baker H (1986) The skin as a barrier. In: Rock A ed. Textbook of dermatology. Oxford, Blackwell Scientific, pp 355–365.

Barker N, Hadgraft J & Rutter N (1987) Skin permeability in the newborn. J Invest Dermatol, **88**(4): 409–411.

Barratt MD (1995a) Quantitative structure–activity relationships for skin permeability. Toxicol In Vitro, **9**(1): 27–37.

Barratt MD (1995b) Quantitative structure activity relationships for skin corrosivity of organic acids, bases and phenols. Toxicol Lett, **75**(1–3): 169–176.

Barry BW (1983) Dermatological formulations: percutaneous absorption. New York, Marcel Dekker (Drugs and the Pharmaceutical Sciences Vol. 18).

Barry BW (1991) The LPP theory of skin penetration enhancement. In: Bronaugh RL & Maibach HI eds. In vitro percutaneous absorption: principles, fundamentals, and applications. Boca Raton, FL, CRC Press, pp 165–185.

Bartek MJ, LaBudde JA & Maibach HI (1972) Skin permeability in vivo: comparison in rat, rabbit, pig and man. J Invest Dermatol, **58**: 114–123.

Bashir SJ, Chew AL, Anigbogu A, Dreher F & Maibach HI (2001) Physical and physiological effects of stratum corneum tape stripping. Skin Res Technol, **7**(1): 40–48.

Baynes RE & Riviere JE (2004) Mixture additives inhibit the dermal permeation of the fatty acid, ricinoleic acid. Toxicol Lett, **147**(1): 15–26.

Beck H, Bracher M & Bartnik FG (1994) Percutaneous absorption of hair dyes: an interlaboratory comparison of in vivo and in vitro data with rat and pig. In Vitro Toxicol, **7**: 305–312.

Benfeldt E (1999) In vivo microdialysis for the investigation of drug levels in the dermis and the effect of barrier perturbation on cutaneous drug penetration. Studies in hairless rats and human subjects. Acta Derm Venereol Suppl (Stockh), **206**: 1–59.

Benfeldt E, Serup J & Menné T (1999) Effect of barrier perturbation on cutaneous salicylic acid penetration in human skin: in vivo pharmacokinetics using microdialysis and non-invasive quantification of barrier function. Br J Dermatol, **140**(4): 739–748.

Benford DJ, Cocker J, Sartorelli P, Schneide T, van Hemmen J & Firth JG (1999) Dermal route in systemic exposure. Scand J Work Environ Health, **25**: 511–520.

Bennat C & Muller-Goymann CC (2000) Skin penetration and stabilization of formulations containing microfine titanium dioxide as physical UV filter. Int J Cosmet Sci, **22**(4): 271–283.

Benson HA (2005) Transdermal drug delivery: penetration enhancement techniques. Curr Drug Deliv, **2**(1): 23–33.

Berner B & Cooper ER (1984) Application of diffusion theory to the relationship between partition coefficient and biological response. J Pharm Sci, **73**(1): 102–106.

Blank IH, Scheuplein RJ & Macfarlane DJ (1967) Mechanism of percutaneous absorption. III. The effect of temperature on the transport of non-electrolytes across the skin. J Invest Dermatol, **49**(6): 582–589.

Blundell G, Henderson WJ & Price EW (1989) Soil particles in the tissues of the foot in endemic elephantiasis of the lower legs. Ann Trop Med Parasitol, **83**: 381–385.

Boehnlein J, Sakr A, Lichtin JL & Bronaugh RL (1994) Characterization of esterase and alcohol dehydrogenase activity in skin. Metabolism of retinyl palmitate to retinol (vitamin A) during percutaneous absorption. Pharm Res, **11**(8): 1155–1159.

Bond JR & Barry BW (1988a) Limitations of hairless mouse skin as a model for in vitro permeation studies through human skin: hydration damage. J Invest Dermatol, **90**(4): 486–489.

Bond JR & Barry BW (1988b) Hairless mouse skin is limited as a model for assessing the effects of penetration enhancers in human skin. J Invest Dermatol, **90**(6): 810–813.

Borgia SL, Regehly M, Sivaramakrishnan R, Mehnert W, Korting HC, Danker K, Roeder B, Kramer KD & Schaefer-Korting M (2005) Lipid nanoparticles for skin penetration enhancement — correlation to drug localization within the particle matrix as determined by fluorescence and parelectric spectroscopy. J Control Release, **110**(1): 151–163.

Bos JD & Meinardi MM (2000) The 500 dalton rule for the skin penetration of chemical compounds and drugs. Exp Dermatol, **9**(3): 165–169.

Bos PJ, Brouwer D, Stevenson H, Boogaard P, de Kort WA & van Hemmen J (1998) Proposal for the assessment of quantitative dermal exposure limits in occupational environments: Part 1. Development of a concept to derive a quantitative dermal occupational exposure limit. Occup Environ Med, **55**(12): 795–804.

Bouwstra J, Pilgram G, Gooris G, Koerten H & Ponec M (2001) New aspects of the skin barrier organization. Skin Pharmacol Appl Skin Physiol, **14**(Suppl. 1): 52–62.

Bouwstra JA, Honeywell-Nguyen PL, Gooris GS & Ponec M (2003a) Structure of the skin barrier and its modulation by vesicular formulations. Prog Lipid Res, **42**(1): 1–36.

Bouwstra JA, de Graaff A, Gooris GS, Nijsse J, Wiechers JW & van Aelst AC (2003b) Water distribution and related morphology in human stratum corneum at different hydration levels. J Invest Dermatol, **120**(5): 750–758.

Brain KR, James VJ & Walters KA eds (1993) Prediction of percutaneous penetration. Vol 3b. Cardiff, STS Publishing (ISBN 0 948917 06 7).

Brain KR, James VJ & Walters KA eds (1996) Prediction of percutaneous penetration. Vol. 4b. Cardiff, STS Publishing (ISBN 0 948917 10 5).

Brain KR, Walters KA & Watkinson AC (1998a) Investigation of skin permeation in vitro. In: Roberts MS & Walters KA eds. Dermal absorption and toxicity assessment. New York, Marcel Dekker, pp 161–187 (Drugs and the Pharmaceutical Sciences Vol. 91).

Brain KR, James VJ & Walters KA eds (1998b) Perspectives in percutaneous penetration. Vol. 5b. Cardiff, STS Publishing (ISBN 0 948917 12 1).

Brain KR, Walters KA, Green DM, Brain S, Loretz LJ, Sharma RK & Dressler WE (2005) Percutaneous penetration of diethanolamine through human skin in vitro: application from cosmetic vehicles. Food Chem Toxicol, **43**(5): 681–690.

Bronaugh RL (1991) A flow-through diffusion cell. In: Bronaugh RL & Maibach HI eds. In vitro percutaneous absorption: principles, fundamentals, and applications. Boca Raton, FL, CRC Press, pp 17–23.

Bronaugh RL (2004a) Methods for in vitro skin metabolism studies. In: Zhai H & Maibach HI eds. Dermatotoxicology, 6th ed. New York, CRC Press, pp 622–630.

Bronaugh RL (2004b) Methods for in vitro percutaneous absorption. In: Zhai H & Maibach HI eds. Dermatotoxicology, 6th ed. New York, CRC Press, pp 520–526.

Bronaugh RL & Congdon ER (1984) Percutaneous absorption of hair dyes: correlation with partition coefficients. J Invest Dermatol, **83**(2): 124–127.

Bronaugh RL & Franz TJ (1986) Vehicle effects on percutaneous absorption: in vivo and in vitro comparisons with human skin. Br J Dermatol, **115**(1): 1–11.

Bronaugh RL & Maibach HI (1985) Percutaneous absorption of nitroaromatic compounds: in vivo and in vitro studies in the human and monkey. J Invest Dermatol, **84**(3): 180–183.

Bronaugh RL & Stewart RF (1984) Methods for in vitro percutaneous absorption studies III: hydrophobic compounds. J Pharm Sci, **73**: 1255–1258.

Bronaugh RL & Stewart RF (1985) Methods for in vitro percutaneous absorption studies IV: the flow-through diffusion cell. J Pharm Sci, **74**: 64–67.

Bronaugh RL, Stewart R, Congdon E & Giles AJ (1982) Methods for in vitro percutaneous absorption studies. I. Comparison with in vivo results. Toxicol Appl Pharmacol, **62**(3): 474–480.

Bronaugh RL, Stewart RF & Simon M (1986) Methods for in vitro percutaneous absorption studies. VIII: Use of excised human skin. J Pharm Sci, **75**(11): 1094–1097.

Bronaugh RL, Hood HL, Kraeling MEK & Yourick JJ (1999) Determination of percutaneous absorption by in vitro techniques. In: Bronaugh RL & Maibach HI eds. Percutaneous absorption: drugs–cosmetics–mechanisms–methodology, 3rd ed. New York, Marcel Dekker, pp 229–233 (Drugs and the Pharmaceutical Sciences Vol. 97).

Brooke I, Cocker J, Delic JI, Payne M, Jones K, Gregg NC & Dyne D (1998) Dermal uptake of solvents from the vapour phase: an experimental study in humans. Ann Occup Hyg, **42**(8): 531–540.

Bucks DAW, Maibach HI & Guy RH (1985) Percutaneous absorption of steroids: effect of repeated application. J Pharm Sci, **74**: 1337–1339.

Bucks D, Guy R & Maibach H (1991) Effects of occlusion. In: Bronaugh RL & Maibach HI eds. In vitro percutaneous absorption: principles, fundamentals, and applications. Boca Raton, FL, CRC Press, pp 85–114.

Bunge AL & Cleek RL (1995) A new method for estimating dermal absorption from chemical exposure: 2. Effect of molecular weight and octanol–water partitioning. Pharm Res, **12**(1): 88–95.

Bunge A & McDougal J (1999) Dermal uptake. In: Olin SS ed. Exposure to contaminants in drinking water: estimating uptake through the skin and by inhalation. Boca Raton, FL, CRC Press, pp 137–181.

Bunge AL & Parks JM (1998) Soil contamination: theoretical descriptions. In: Roberts MS & Walters KA eds. Dermal absorption and toxicity assessment. New York, Marcel Dekker, pp 669–696.

Bunge AL, Cleek RL & Vecchia BE (1995) A new method for estimating dermal absorption from chemical exposure. 3. Compared with steady-state methods for prediction and data analysis. Pharm Res, **12**(7): 972–982.

Bunge AL, Tourailee GD, Marty JP & Guy RH (2005) Modelling dermal absorption from soils and powders using stratum corneum tape-stripping in vivo. In: Riviere JE ed. Dermal absorption models in toxicology and pharmacology. Boca Raton, FL, Taylor & Francis, pp 191–212.

Cabral-Lilly D & Walters K (2004) Novel dual therapy — physicochemical strategies for treating psoriasis. In: Brain KR & Walters KA eds. Perspectives in percutaneous penetration. Vol. 9a. Abstracts of presentations at the ninth international perspectives in percutaneous penetration conference held in La Grande Motte, April 2004. Cardiff, STS Publishing, p 17.

Chao YC & Nylander-French LA (2004) Determination of keratin protein in a tape-stripped skin sample from jet fuel exposed skin. Ann Occup Hyg, **48**(1): 65–73.

Chen C & Sartorelli P (2005) Proceedings of the international conference on occupational and environmental exposures of skin to chemicals: science and policy — session II: health effects and hazard identification. Regul Toxicol Pharmacol, **41**(2): 150–158.

Chilcott RP, Barai N, Beezer AE, Brain SI, Brown MB, Bunge AL, Burgess SE, Cross S, Dalton CH, Dias M, Farinha A, Finnin BC, Gallagher SJ, Green DM, Gunt H, Gwyther RL, Heard CM, Jarvis CA, Kamiyama F, Kasting GB, Ley EE, Lim ST, McNaughton GS, Morris A, Nazemi MH, Pellett MA, du Plessis J, Quan YS, Raghavan SL, Roberts M, Romonchuk W, Roper CS, Schenk D, Simonsen L, Simpson A, Traversa BD, Trottet L, Watkinson A, Wilkinson SC, Williams FM, Yamamoto A & Hadgraft J (2005) Inter- and intralaboratory variation of in vitro diffusion cell measurements: an international multicenter study using quasi-standardized methods and materials. J Pharm Sci, **94**(3): 632–638.

Choi EH, Brown BE, Crumrine D, Chang S, Man MQ, Elias PM & Feingold KR (2005) Mechanisms by which psychologic stress alters cutaneous permeability barrier homeostasis and stratum corneum integrity. J Invest Dermatol, **124**(3): 587–595.

Choi MJ, Zhai H & Maibach HI (2004) Tape stripping method and stratum corneum. In: Zhai H & Maibach HI eds. Dermatotoxicology. Boca Raton, FL, CRC Press, pp 533–548.

Chu I, Dick D, Bronaugh R & Tryphonas L (1996) Skin reservoir formation and bioavailability of dermally administered chemicals in hairless guinea pigs. Food Chem Toxicol, **34**: 267–276.

Clark NW, Scott RC, Blain PG & Williams FM (1993) Fate of fluazifop butyl in rat and human skin in vitro. Arch Toxicol, **67**(1): 44–48.

Cleek RL & Bunge AL (1993) A new method for estimating dermal absorption from chemical exposure. 1. General approach. Pharm Res, **10**(4): 497–506.

Clowes HM, Scott RC & Heylings JR (1994) Skin absorption: Flow-through or static diffusion cells. Toxicol In Vitro, **8**: 827–830.

Cnubben NH, Elliott GR, Hakkert BC, Meuling WJ & van de Sandt JJ (2002) Comparative in vitro–in vivo percutaneous penetration of the fungicide *ortho*-phenylphenol. Regul Toxicol Pharmacol, **35**: 198–208.

Collier SW, Sheikh NM, Sakr A, Lichtin JL, Stewart RF & Bronaugh RL (1989) Maintenance of skin viability during in vitro percutaneous absorption/metabolism studies. Toxicol Appl Pharmacol, **99**: 522–533.

Collier S, Storm J & Bronaugh R (1993) Reduction of azo dyes during in vitro percutaneous absorption. Toxicol Appl Pharmacol, **118**: 73–79.

Cooper CS, Vigny P, Kindts M, Grover PL & Sims P (1980) Metabolic activation of 3-methylcholanthrene in mouse skin: fluorescence spectral evidence indicates the involvement of diol-epoxides formed in the 7,8,9,10-ring. Carcinogenesis, **1**(10): 855–860.

Coquette A, Berna N, Poumay Y & Pittelkow MR (2000) The keratinocyte in cutaneous irritation and sensitisation. In: Kydonieus AF & Wille JJ eds. Biochemical modulation of skin reactions: transdermals, tropicals, cosmetics. Boca Raton, FL, CRC Press, pp 125–143.

Corachan M, Tura JM, Campo E, Soley M & Traveria A (1988) Podoconiosis in Equatorial Guinea. Report of two cases from different geological environments. Trop Geogr Med, **40**: 359–364.

Corish J (2004) Modelling percutaneous penetration. In: Brain KR & Walters KA eds. Perspectives in percutaneous penetration. Vol. 9a. Abstracts of presentations at the ninth international perspectives in percutaneous penetration conference held in La Grande Motte, April 2004. Cardiff, STS Publishing, p 9.

Corish J, Golden D, Kezic S & Krüse J (2004) Comparative analysis of non-steady state data using two diffusion models. In: Brain KR & Walters KA eds. Perspectives in percutaneous penetration. Vol. 9a. Abstracts of presentations at the ninth international perspectives in percutaneous penetration conference held in La Grande Motte, April 2004. Cardiff, STS Publishing, p 95.

Crank J (1975) The mathematics of diffusion. Oxford, Clarendon Press.

Cronin MTD & Schultz TW (2001) Development of quantitative structure–activity relationships for the toxicity of aromatic compounds to *Tetrahymena pyriformis*: comparative assessment of the methodologies. Chem Res Toxicol, **14**: 1284–1295.

Cronin MTD, Dearden JC, Moss GP & Murray-Dickson G (1999) Investigation of the mechanism of flux across human skin in vitro by quantitative structure–permeability relationships. Eur J Pharm Sci, **7**: 325–330.

Cross SE & Roberts MS (1999) Defining a model to predict the distribution of topically applied growth factors and other solutes in excisional full-thickness wounds. J Invest Dermatol, **112**(1): 36–41.

Cross SE & Roberts MS (2000) The effect of occlusion on epidermal penetration of parabens from a commercial allergy test ointment, acetone and ethanol vehicles. J Invest Dermatol, **115**(5): 914–918.

Cross SE & Roberts MS (2005) Effects of dermal blood flow, lymphatics and binding as determinants of topical absorption, clearance and distribution. In: Riviere JE ed. Dermal absorption models in toxicology and pharmacology. Boca Raton, FL, Taylor & Francis, pp 249–279.

Cross SE, Anderson C, Thompson MJ & Roberts MS (1997) Is there tisuse penetration after application of topical salicylate formulations? Lancet, **350**(9078): 636.

Cross SE, Anderson C & Roberts MS (1998) Topical penetration of commercial salicylate esters and salts using human isolated skin and clinical microdialysis studies. Br J Clin Pharmacol, **46**(1): 29–35.

Cussler EL (1997) Diffusion: mass transfer in fluid systems. Cambridge, Cambridge University Press.

Daston G, Faustman E, Ginsberg G, Fenner-Crisp P, Olin S, Sonawane B, Bruckner J & Breslin W (2004) A framework for assessing risks to children from exposure to environmental agents. Environ Health Perspect, **112**(2): 238–256.

Davaran S, Rashidi MR & Hashemi M (2003) Synthesis and hydrolytic behaviour of 2-mercaptoethyl ibuprofenate–polyethylene glycol conjugate as a novel transdermal prodrug. J Pharm Pharmacol, **55**(4): 513–517.

Davies DJ, Ward RJ & Heylings JR (2004) Multi-species assessment of electrical resistance as a skin integrity marker for in vitro percutaneous absorption studies. Toxicol In Vitro, **18**(3): 351–358.

Davis AF & Hadgraft J (1991) Effect of supersaturation on membrane transport: 1. Hydrocortisone acetate. Int J Pharm, **76**: 1–8.

Davis AF, Gyurik RJ, Hadgraft J, Pellett MA & Walters KA (2002) Formulation strategies for modulating skin permeation. In: Walters KA ed. Dermatological and transdermal formulations. New York, Marcel Dekker, pp 271–317 (Drugs and the Pharmaceutical Sciences Vol. 119).

Dearden JC, Cronin MTD, Patel H & Raevsky OA (2000) QSAR prediction of human skin permeability coefficients. J Pharm Pharmacol, **52**(Suppl.): 221.

Degim IT, Pugh WJ & Hadgraft J (1998) Skin permeability data: anomalous results. Int J Pharm, **170**: 129–133.

Degim T, Hadgraft J, Ilbasmis S & Oezkan Y (2003) Prediction of skin penetration using artificial neural network (ANN) modeling. J Pharm Sci, **92**(3): 656–664.

Dehghanyar P, Mayer BX, Namiranian K, Mascher H, Müller M & Brunner M (2004) Topical skin penetration of diclofenac after single- and multiple-dose application. Int J Clin Pharmacol Ther Toxicol, **42**(7): 353–359.

de Jager MW, Gooris GS, Dolbnya IP, Bras W, Ponec M & Bouwstra JA (2003) The phase behaviour of skin lipid mixtures based on synthetic ceramides. Chem Phys Lipids, **124**(2): 123–134.

de Jager MW, Gooris GS, Dolbnya IP, Bras W, Ponec M & Bouwstra JA (2004) Novel lipid mixtures based on synthetic ceramides reproduce the unique stratum corneum lipid organization. J Lipid Res, **45**(5): 923–932.

Dick IP, Blain PG & Williams FM (1997a) The percutaneous absorption and skin distribution of lindane in man. I. In vivo studies. Hum Exp Toxicol, **16**(11): 645–651.

Dick IP, Blain PG & Williams FM (1997b) The percutaneous absorption and skin distribution of lindane in man. II. In vitro studies. Hum Exp Toxicol, **16**(11): 652–657.

Dickel H, Bruckner TM, Erdmann SM, Fluhr JW, Frosch PJ, Grabbe J, Loffler H, Merk HF, Pirker C, Schwanitz HJ, Weisshaar E & Brasch J (2004) The "strip" patch test: results of a multicentre study towards a standardization. Arch Dermatol Res, **296**(5): 212–219.

Diembeck W, Beck H, Benech-Kieffer F, Courtellemont P, Dupuis J, Lovell W, Paye M, Spengler J & Steiling W (1999) Test guidelines for in vitro assessment of dermal absorption and percutaneous penetration of cosmetic ingredients. European Cosmetic, Toiletry and Perfumery Association. Food Chem Toxicol, **37**(2–3): 191–205.

Donahue JM (1996) Memorandum from J.M. Donahue, Chief, Worker Health and Safety Branch, State of California, to G. Patterson, Chief Medical Toxicology Branch, 5 July 1996, HSM-96005. Revised policy on dermal absorption default for pesticides. 2 pp.

Donnelly RF, McCarron PA & Woolfson AD (2005) Drug delivery of aminolevulinic acid from topical formulations intended for photodynamic therapy. Photochem Photobiol, **81**(4): 750–767.

Dressler WE (1999) Hair dye absorption. In: Bronaugh RL & Maibach HI eds. Percutaneous absorption: drugs–cosmetics–mechanisms–methodology, 3rd ed. New York, Marcel Dekker, pp 685–716 (Drugs and the Pharmaceutical Sciences Vol. 97).

Drexler H (1998) Assignment of skin notation for MAK values and its legal consequences in Germany. Int Arch Occup Environ Health, **71**: 503–505.

Dugard PH (1977) Skin permeability theory in relation to measurements of percutaneous absorption in toxicology. In: Marzulli FN & Maibach HI eds. Dermatotoxicology and pharmacology. Washington, DC, Hemisphere Publishing Corp., pp 525–550 (Advances in Modern Toxicology Vol. 4).

Dugard PH & Scott RC (1984) Absorption through skin. In: Baden HP ed. Chemotherapy of psoriasis. Oxford, Pergamon Press, pp 125–144.

Dugard PH, Walker M, Mawdsley SJ & Scott RC (1984) Absorption of some glycol ethers through human skin in vitro. Environ Health Perspect, **57**: 193–197.

Dupuis D, Rougier A, Roguet R, Lotte C & Kalopissis G (1984) In vivo relationship between horny layer reservoir effect and percutaneous absorption in human and rat. J Invest Dermatol, **82**: 353–358.

Dutkiewicz T & Piotrowski J (1961) Experimental investigations on the quantitative estimation of aniline absorption in man. Pure Appl Chem, **3**: 319–323.

Dutkiewicz T & Tyras H (1967) A study of the skin absorption of ethylbenzene in man. Br J Ind Med, **24**: 330–332.

Dutkiewicz T & Tyras H (1968) Skin absorption of toluene, styrene, and xylene by man. Br J Ind Med, **25**(3): 243.

Dutkiewicz T, Baranowska-Dutkiewicz B & Konczalik J (2000) Percutaneous absorption studies after forty years. Int J Occup Environ Health, **6**(2): 111–113.

EC (2001) Draft guidance document. Guidance for the setting of acceptable operator exposure levels (AOELs). European Commisson, pp 1–16 (7531/VI/95 rev. 6; http://europa.eu.int/comm/food/plant/protection/resources/7531_vi_95.pdf).

EC (2003) Technical guidance document (TGD) in support of Commission Directive 93/67/EEC on risk assessment for new notified substances. European Commission, Part 1, pp 1–303 (http://ecb.jrc.it/technical-guidance-document/).

EC (2004) Guidance document on dermal absorption. European Commission, pp 1–15 (Sanco/222/2000 rev. 7; http://www.eu.int/comm/food/plant/protection/evaluation/guidance/wrkdoc20_rev_en.pdf).

ECETOC (1993) Percutaneous absorption. Brussels, European Centre for Ecotoxicology and Toxicology of Chemicals, pp 1–80 (Monograph No. 20).

EDETOX (2004) Quality of life and management of living resources. Final report for dissemination. European Commission, Evaluation and Predictions of Dermal Absorption of Toxic Chemicals, 61 pp (Contract No. QLK4-2000-00196; http://www.ncl.ac.uk/edetox/currentposition.html).

EDETOX (undated) Evaluations and Predictions of Dermal Absorption of Toxic Chemicals website. European Union Framework V: Quality of Life, Environment and Health Key Action Funding (Project No. QLKA-2000-00196; http://www.ncl.ac.uk/edetox).

Elias PM (1981) Epidermal lipids, membranes, and keratinization. Int J Dermatol, **20**(1): 1–19.

El Marbouh L, Arellano C, Philibert C, Evrard P, Poey J & Houin G (2000) In vivo study of percutaneous absorption of 4-chloroaniline using microdialysis in the rat. Arzneimittel-forschung, **50**(11): 1033–1036.

Eppler AR, Kraeling ME, Wickett RR & Bronaugh RL (2005) Percutaneous absorption, metabolism, and irritation potential of arachidonic acid and glyceryl arachidonate using in vitro diffusion cell techniques. Society of Cosmetic Chemists Annual Scientific Seminar Abstracts.

Feldmann RJ & Maibach HI (1967) Regional variation in percutaneous penetration of ^{14}C cortisol in man. J Invest Dermatol, **48**: 181–183.

Feldmann RJ & Maibach IR (1969) Percutaneous penetration of steroids in man. J Invest Dermatol, **52**(1): 89–94.

Feldmann RJ & Maibach IH (1970) Absorption of some organic compounds through the skin in man. J Invest Dermatol, **54**(5): 399–404.

Feldmann RJ & Maibach HI (1974) Percutaneous penetration of some pesticides and herbicides in man. Toxicol Appl Pharmacol, **28**: 126–132.

Fiserova-Bergerova V, Pierce J & Droz P (1990) Dermal absorption potential of industrial chemicals: Criteria for skin notation. Am J Ind Med, **17**: 617–635.

Fitzpatrick D, Corish J & Hayes B (2004) Modelling skin permeability for risk assessment — the future. Chemosphere, **55**: 1309–1314.

Fluhr JW, Lazzerini S, Distante F, Gloor M & Berardesca E (1999) Effects of prolonged occlusion on stratum corneum barrier function and water holding capacity. Skin Pharmacol Appl Skin Physiol, **12**(4): 193–198.

Flynn GL (1985) Mechanism of percutaneous absorption from physicochemical evidence. In: Bronough RL & Maibach HI eds. Percutaneous absorption: mechanisms–methodology–drug delivery. New York, Marcel Dekker, pp 17–42.

Flynn GL (1990) Physicochemical determinants of skin absorption. In: Gerrity TR & Henry CJ eds. Principles of route-to-route extrapolation for risk assessment. New York, Elsevier, pp 93–127.

Flynn GL & Yalkowsky SH (1972) Correlation and prediction of mass transport across membranes. I. Influence of alkyl chain length on flux-determining properties of barrier and diffusant. J Pharm Sci, **61**(6): 838–852.

Ford RA, Hawkins DR, Mayo BC & Api AM (2001) The in vivo dermal absorption and metabolism of [4-^{14}C] coumarin by rats and by human volunteers under simulated conditions of use in fragrances. Food Chem Toxicol, **39**(2): 153–162.

Franz TJ (1975) Percutaneous absorption. On the relevance of in vitro data. J Invest Dermatol, **64**(3): 190–195.

Franz TJ (1978) The finite dose technique as a valid in vitro model for the study of percutaneous absorption in man. Curr Probl Dermatol, **7**: 58–68.

Frasch HF & Landsittel DP (2002) Regarding the sources of data analyzed with quantitative structure–skin permeability relationship methods [commentary on "Investigation of the mechanism of flux across human skin in vitro by quantitative structure–permeability relationship", Eur J Pharm Sci 1999 Mar;7(4):325–330]. Eur J Pharm Sci, **15**(5): 399–403.

Friend DR (1992) In vitro skin permeation techniques. J Control Release, **18**: 235–248.

Garfitt SJ, Jones K, Mason HJ & Cocker J (2002a) Oral and dermal exposure to propetamphos: a human volunteer study. Toxicol Lett, **134**(1–3): 115–118.

Garfitt SJ, Jones K, Mason HJ & Cocker J (2002b) Exposure to the organophosphate diazinon: data from a human volunteer study with oral and dermal doses. Toxicol Lett, **134**(1–3): 105–113.

Garfitt SJ, Jones K, Mason HJ & Cocker J (2002c) Development of a urinary biomarker for exposure to the organophosphate propetamphos: data from an oral and dermal human volunteer study. Biomarkers, **7**(2): 113–122.

Geinoz S, Guy RH, Testa B & Carrupt PA (2004) Quantitative structure–permeation relationships (QSPeRs) to predict skin permeation: a critical evaluation. Pharm Res, **21**(1): 83–91.

Gerner I, Barratt MD, Zinke S, Schlegel K & Schlede E (2004) Development and prevalidation of a list of structure–activity relationship rules to be used in expert systems for prediction of the skin-sensitising properties of chemicals. Altern Lab Anim, **32**(5): 487–509.

Golden D, Fitzpatrick D & Corish J (2004) QSARs for percutaneous penetration. In: Brain KR & Walters KA eds. Perspectives in percutaneous penetration. Vol. 9a. Abstracts of presentations at the ninth international perspectives in percutaneous penetration conference held in La Grande Motte, April 2004. Cardiff, STS Publishing, p 94.

Gordon Research Conference (2005) Gordon Research Conference on Barrier Function of Mammalian Skin, 7–12 August 2005, Mount Molyoke College, South Hadley, MA (http://www.grc.uri.edu/programs/2005/barrier.htm).

Gould AR, Sharp PJ, Smith DR, Stegink AJ, Chase CJ, Kovacs JC, Penglis S, Chatterton BE & Bunn CL (2003) Increased permeability of psoriatic skin to the protein, plasminogen activator inhibitor 2. Arch Dermatol Res, **295**(6): 249–254.

Grissom RE, Brownie C & Guthrie FE (1987) In vivo and in vitro dermal penetration of lipophilic and hydrophilic pesticides in mice. Bull Environ Contam Toxicol, **38**: 917–924.

Grubauer G, Feingold KR & Elias PM (1987) Relationship of epidermal lipogenesis to cutaneous barrier function. J Lipid Res, **28**(6): 746–752.

Guillot M (1954) Physiochemical conditions of cutaneous absorption. J Physiol, **46**: 31–49.

Gupta E, Wientjes MG & Au JL (1995) Penetration kinetics of 2',3'-dideoxyinosine in dermis is described by the distributed model. Pharm Res, **12**(1): 108–112.

Gute BD, Grunwald GD & Basak SC (1999) Prediction of the dermal penetration of polycyclic aromatic hydrocarbons (PAHs): a hierarchical QSAR approach. SAR QSAR Environ Res, **10**: 1–15.

Hadgraft J & Valenta C (2000) pH, pK_a and dermal delivery. Int J Pharm, **200**: 243–247.

Hadgraft JD, Beutner D & Wolff HM (1993) In vivo–in vitro comparisons in the transdermal delivery of nitroglycerin. Int J Pharm, **89**(1): R1–R4.

Hakkert BC, van de Sandt JJM, Bessems JGM & de Heer C (2005) Dermal absorption of pesticides. In: Franklin CA & Worgan JP eds. Occupational and residential exposure assessment for pesticides. Chichester, Wiley Publishers, pp 319–345.

Hanke J, Dutkiewicz T & Piotrowski J (1961) Cutaneous absorption of benzene vapors in man. Med Pr, **12**: 413–426.

Hanke J, Dutkiewicz T & Piotrowski J (2000) The absorption of benzene through human skin. Int J Occup Environ Health, **6**(2): 104–111.

Haselbeck RJ, Ang HL & Duester G (1997) Class IV alcohol/retinol dehydrogenase localization in epidermal basal layer: potential site of retinoic acid synthesis during skin development. Dev Dynam, **208**: 447–453.

Hata M, Tokura Y, Takigawa M, Sato M, Shioya Y, Fujikura Y & Imokawa G (2002) Assessment of epidermal barrier function by photoacoustic spectrometry in relation to its importance in the pathogenesis of atopic dermatitis. Lab Invest, **82**(11): 1451–1461.

Hatsell S & Cowin P (2001) Deconstructing desmoplakin. Nat Cell Biol, **3**: E270–E272.

Hawkins DR, Elsom LF, Kirkpatrick D, Ford RA & Api AM (2002) Dermal absorption and disposition of musk ambrette, musk ketone and musk xylene in human subjects. Toxicol Lett, **131**(3): 147–151.

Hewitt PG, Perkins J & Hotchkiss SA (2000) Metabolism of fluroxypyr, fluroxypyr methyl ester, and the herbicide fluroxypyr methylheptyl ester. II: In rat skin homogenates. Drug Metab Dispos, **28**(7): 755–759.

Heylings JR, van de Sandt JJM, Gilde AJ & Ward RJ (2001) Evaluation of SkinEthic human reconstituted epidermis for percutaneous absorption testing. Toxicology, **164**: 130 (Abstract P2F1).

Higuchi TJ (1960) Physical chemical analysis of percutaneous absorption process from creams and ointments. J Soc Cosmet Chem, **11**: 85–87.

Hinz RS, Lorence CR, Hodson CD, Hansch C, Hall LL & Guy RH (1991) Percutaneous penetration of *para*-substituted phenols in vitro. Fundam Appl Toxicol, **17**(3): 575–583.

Hood HL, Wickett RR & Bronaugh RL (1996) In vitro percutaneous absorption of the fragrance ingredient musk xylol. Food Chem Toxicol, **34**(5): 483–488.

Hostynek JJ (2003) Factors determining percutaneous metal absorption. Food Chem Toxicol, **41**(3): 327–345.

Hostynek JJ & Magee PS (1997) Modelling in vivo human skin absorption. Quant Struct Act Relat, **16**: 473–479.

Hostynek J, Hinz RS, Lorence CR & Guy RH (1998) Human skin penetration by metal compounds. In: Roberts MS & Walters KA eds. Dermal absorption and toxicity assessment. New York, Marcel Dekker, pp 647–668 (Drugs and the Pharmaceutical Sciences Vol. 91).

Hotchkiss SAM (1995) Cutaneous toxicity: kinetic and metabolic determinants. Toxicol Ecotoxicol, **2**(1): 10–18.

Hotchkiss SAM (1998) Dermal metabolism. In: Roberts MS & Walter KA eds. Dermal absorption and toxicity assessment. New York, Marcel Dekker, pp 43–101 (Drug and the Pharmaceutical Sciences Vol. 91).

Hotchkiss SA, Chidgey MAJ, Rose S & Caldwell J (1990) Percutaneous absorption of benzyl acetate through rat skin in vitro. 1. Validation of an in vitro model against in vivo data. Food Chem Toxicol, **28**: 443–447.

Howes D, Guy R, Hadgraft J, Heylings J, Hoeck U, Kemper F, Maibach H, Marty J-P, Merk H, Parra J, Rekkas D, Rondelli I, Schaefer H, Täuber U & Verbiese N (1996) Methods for assessing percutaneous absorption. Altern Lab Anim, **24**: 81–106.

Hughes MF, Shrivastava SP, Fisher HL & Hall LL (1993) Comparative in vitro percutaneous absorption of *p*-substituted phenols through rat skin using static and flow-through diffusion systems. Toxicol In Vitro, **7**(3): 221–227.

Humbert P (2003) [Functional consequences of cutaneous lipid perturbation.] Pathol Biol, **51**(5): 271–274 (in French).

ICH (1996) Guideline for good clinical practice E6(R1). ICH harmonised tripartite guideline. International Conference on Harmonization, pp 1–57 (http://www.ich.org).

Idson B (1971) Biophysical factors in skin penetration. J Soc Cosmet Chem, **22**: 615–634.

Idson B (1975) Percutaneous absorption. J Pharm Sci, **64**(6): 901–924.

Idson B & Behl CR (1987) Drug structure vs penetration. In: Kydonieus AF & Berner B eds. Transdermal delivery of drugs. Boca Raton, FL, CRC Press, pp 85–151.

IPCS (1994) Assessing human health risks of chemicals: Derivation of guidance values for health-based exposure limits. Geneva, World Health Organization, International Programme on Chemical Safety (Environmental Health Criteria 170).

IPCS (2001) Biomarkers in risk assessment. Geneva, World Health Organization, International Programme on Chemical Safety (Environmental Health Criteria 222).

Islam MS, Zhao L, Zhou J, Dong L, McDougal JN & Flynn GL (1999) Systemic uptake and clearance of chloroform by hairless rats following dermal exposure: II. Absorption of the neat solvent. Am Ind Hyg Assoc J, **60**(4): 438–443.

Jakasa I, Kezic S & Calkoen F (2004a) Determination of the percutaneous absorption of polyethylene glycols of different molecular weight in volunteers by tape stripping. In: Brain KR & Walters KA eds. Perspectives in percutaneous penetration. Vol. 9a. Abstracts of presentations at the ninth international perspectives in percutaneous penetration conference held in La Grande Motte, April 2004. Cardiff, STS Publishing, p 97.

Jakasa I, Mohammadi N, Krüse J & Kezic S (2004b) Percutaneous absorption of neat and aqueous solutions of 2-butoxyethanol in volunteers. Int Arch Occup Environ Health, **77**: 79–84.

Jakasa I, Verbeck MM, Esposito M & Kezic S (2005) Differences in percutaneous absorption in normal subjects and atopic dermatitis patients in relation to the molecular weight. In: Proceedings of the second international conference on occupational and environmental exposures of skin to chemicals – 2005, 12–15 June, Stockholm, Sweden. Co-sponsored by the National Institute for Occupational Safety and Health and Karolinska Institutet, Abstract P91, p 161 (http://www.cdc.gov/niosh/topics/skin/OEESC2/authorindex.html).

Jaworska JS, Comber M, Auer C & van Leeuwen CJ (2003) Summary of a workshop on regulatory acceptance of (Q)SARs for human health and environmental endpoints. Environ Health Perspect, **111**: 1358–1360.

Jewell C, Heylings J, Clowes HM & Williams FM (2000) Percutaneous absorption and metabolism of dinitrochlorobenzene in vitro. Arch Toxicol, **74**(7): 356–365.

Johanson G (2003) Dermal absorption and principles for skin notation. In: Occupational exposure limits — approaches and criteria. Proceedings from a Nordic Institute for Advanced Training in Occupational Health (NIVA) course held in Uppsala, Sweden, 24–28 September 2001. Stockholm, National Institute for Working Life, pp 79–86 (Arbete och hälsa 17).

Johanson G (2005) Beyond skin notation — modeling percutaneous absorption. In: Proceedings of the second international conference on occupational and environmental exposures of skin to chemicals – 2005, 12–15 June, Stockholm, Sweden. Co-sponsored by the National Institute for Occupational Safety and Health and Karolinska Institutet, abstract for plenary talk 5.1, pp 20–22 (http://www.cdc.gov/niosh/topics/skin/OEESC2/authorindex.html).

Johanson G & Boman A (1991) Percutaneous absorption of 2-butoxyethanol vapour in human subjects. Br J Ind Med, **48**: 788–792.

Johnson JM, Brengelmann GL, Hales JR, Vanhoutte PM & Wenger CB (1986) Regulation of the cutaneous circulation. Fed Proc, **45**(13): 2841–2850.

Johnson ME, Blankschtein D & Langer R (1995) Permeation of steroids through human skin. J Pharm Sci, **84**(9): 1144–1146.

Jones AD, Dick IP, Cherrie JW, Cronin MTD, van de Sandt JJM, Esdaile DJ, Iyengar S, ten Berge W, Wilkinson SC, Roper CS, Semple S, de Heer C & Williams FM (2004) CEFIC workshop on methods to determine dermal permeation for human risk assessment. European Chemical Industry Council, December, pp 1–86 (Research Report TM/04/07; http://www.iom-world.org/pubs/IOM_TM0407.pdf).

Jones K, Cocker J, Dodd LJ & Fraser I (2003) Factors affecting the extent of dermal absorption of solvent vapours: a human volunteer study. Ann Occup Hyg, **47**(2): 145–150.

Joukhadar C & Muller M (2005) Microdialysis: current applications in clinical pharmacokinetic studies and its potential role in the future. Clin Pharmacokinet, **44**(9): 895–913.

Jung CT, Wickett RR, Desai PB & Bronaugh RL (2003) In vitro and in vivo percutaneous absorption of catechol. Food Chem Toxicol, **41**(6): 885–895.

Kalia YN, Nonato LB, Lund CH & Guy RG (1996) Development of skin barrier function in low birthweight infants. Pharm Res, **13**(9): S382 (Abstract PDD 7598).

Kalinin AE, Kajava AV & Steinert PM (2002) Epithelial barrier function: assembly and structural features of the cornified cell envelope. Bioassays, **24**(9): 789–800.

Kalnas J & Teitelbaum DT (2000) Dermal absorption of benzene: implications for work practices and regulations. Int J Occup Environ Health, **6**(2): 114–121.

Kammerau B, Zesch A & Schaefer H (1975) Absolute concentrations of dithranol and triacetyl-dithranol in the skin layers after local treatment: in vivo investigations with four different types of pharmaceutical vehicles. J Invest Dermatol, **64**(3): 145–149.

Kao J & Carver MP (1990) Cutaneous metabolism of xenobiotics. Drug Metab Rev, **22**: 363–410.

Kao J, Patterson F & Hall L (1985) Skin penetration and metabolism of topically applied chemicals in six mammalian species, including man: an in vitro study with benzo(*a*)pyrene and testosterone. Toxicol Appl Pharmacol, **81**: 502–516.

Kasting GB & Miller MA (2006) Kinetics of finite dose absorption through skin 2: Volatile compounds. J Pharm Sci, **95**(2): 268–280.

Kasting GB & Robinson PJ (1993) Can we assign an upper limit to skin permeability? Pharm Res, **10**(6): 930–931.

Kasting GB & Saiyasombati P (2001) A physico-chemical properties based model for estimating evaporation and absorption rates of perfumes from skin. Int J Cosmet Sci, **23**: 49–58.

Kasting GB, Smith RL & Cooper ER (1987) Effect of lipid solubility and molecular size on percutaneous absorption. In: Shroot B & Schaefer H eds. Skin pharmacokinetics. Basel, Karger, pp 138–153 (Pharmacology and the Skin Vol. 1).

Kasting GB, Francis WR, Bowman LA & Kinnett GO (1997) Percutaneous absorption of vanilloids: in vivo and in vitro studies. J Pharm Sci, **86**(1): 142–146.

Kenyon S, Carmichael PL, Khalaque S, Panchal S, Waring R, Harris R, Smith RL & Mitchell SC (2004a) The passage of trimethylamine across rat and human skin. Food Chem Toxicol, **42**(10): 1619–1628.

Kenyon SH, Bhattacharyya J, Benson CJ & Carmichael PL (2004b) Percutaneous penetration and genotoxicity of 4,4'-methylenedianiline through rat and human skin in vitro. Toxicology, **196**(1–2): 65–75.

Kezic S (2004) Human in vivo studies of dermal penetration, their relation to in vitro prediction. In: Brain KR & Walters KA eds. Perspectives in percutaneous penetration. Vol. 9a. Abstracts of presentations at the ninth international perspectives in percutaneous penetration conference held in La Grande Motte, April 2004. Cardiff, STS Publishing, p 8.

Kezic S, Mahieu K, Monster A & de Wolff F (1997) Dermal absorption of vaporous and liquid 2-methoxyethanol and 2-ethoxyethanol in volunteers. Occup Environ Med, **54**: 38–43.

Kezic S, Monster AC, Krüse J & Verberk MM (2000) Skin absorption of some vaporous solvents in volunteers. Int Arch Occup Environ Health, **73**(6): 415–422.

Kezic S, Monster AC, van de Gevel IA, Kruse J, Opdam JJ & Verberk MM (2001) Dermal absorption of neat liquid solvents on brief exposures in volunteers. AIHA J (Fairfax, Va) **62**(1): 12–18.

Kezic S, Janmaat A, Krüse J, Monster AC & Verberk MM (2004) Percutaneous absorption of *m*-xylene vapour in volunteers during pre-steady and steady state. Toxicol Lett, **153**(2): 273–282.

Kim S, Lim YT, Soltesz EG, De Grand AM, Lee J, Nakayama A, Parker JA, Mihaljevic T, Laurence RG, Dor DM, Cohn LH, Bawendi MG & Frangioni JV (2004) Near-infrared fluorescent type II quantum dots for sentinel lymph node mapping. Nat Biotechnol, **22**(1): 93–97.

Kirchner LA, Moody RP, Doyle E, Bose R, Jeffrey J & Chu I (1997) The prediction of skin permeability by using physicochemical data. Altern Lab Anim, **25**: 359–370.

Klain GJ & Reifenrath WG (1991) In vivo assessment of dermal absorption. In: Hobson DW ed. Dermal and ocular toxicology — Fundaments and methods. London, CRC Press, pp 247–266.

Kligman AM (1983) A biological brief on percutaneous absorption. Drug Dev Ind Pharm, **9**(4): 521–560.

Kohli AK & Alpar HO (2004) Potential use of nanoparticles for transcutaneous vaccine delivery: effect of particle size and charge. Int J Pharm, **275**: 13–17.

Korinth G, Wellner T, Jakasa I, Kezic S, Krüse J & Schaller KH (2004) Assessment of percutaneous absorption of 2-butoxyethanol by microdialysis in volunteers. In: Brain KR & Walters KA eds. Perspectives in percutaneous penetration. Vol. 9a. Abstracts of presentations at the ninth international perspectives in percutaneous penetration conference held in La Grande Motte, April 2004. Cardiff, STS Publishing, p 100.

Kraeling MEK, Lipicky RJ & Bronaugh RL (1996) Metabolism of benzocaine during percutaneous absorption in the hairless guinea pig: Acetylbenzocaine formation and activity. Skin Pharmacol, **9**: 221–230.

Kraeling ME, Yourick JJ & Bronaugh RL (2004) In vitro human skin penetration of diethanolamine. Food Chem Toxicol, **42**(10): 1553–1561.

Kranz G, Schaefer H & Zesch A (1977) Hydrocortisone (cortisol) concentration and penetration gradient. Acta Derm Venereol, **57**(3): 269–273.

Kretsos K & Kasting GB (2005) Dermal capillary clearance: physiology and modeling. Skin Pharmacol Physiol, **18**(2): 55–74.

Kretsos K, Kasting GB & Nitsche JM (2004) Distributed diffusion–clearance model for transient drug distribution within the skin. J Pharm Sci, **93**(11): 2820–2835.

Kromhout H, Fransman W, Vermeulen R, Roff M & van Hemmen JJ (2004) Variability of task-based dermal exposure measurements from a variety of workplaces. Ann Occup Hyg, **48**(3): 187–196.

Krüse J & Kezic S (2004) Interpretation and extrapolation of dermal permeation data using a mechanistically based mathematical model. In: Brain KR & Walters KA eds. Perspectives in percutaneous penetration. Vol. 9a. Abstracts of presentations at the ninth international perspectives in percutaneous penetration conference held in La Grande Motte, April 2004. Cardiff, STS Publishing, p 96.

Lademann J, Weigmann H, Rickmeyer C, Barthelmes H, Schaefer H, Mueller G, Sterry W (1999) Penetration of titanium dioxide microparticles in a sunscreen formulation into the horny layer and the follicular orifice. Skin Pharmacol Appl Skin Physiol, **12**: 247–256.

Lademann J, Otberg N, Richter H, Weigmann HJ, Lindemann U, Schaefer H, Sterry W (2001) Investigation of follicular penetration of topically applied substances. Skin Pharmacol Appl Skin Physiol, **14**: 17–22.

Lansdown ABG & Taylor A (1997) Zinc and titanium oxides: promising UV-absorbers but what influence do they have on the intact skin? Int J Cosmet Sci, **19**(4): 167–172.

Larese Filon F, Maina G, Adami G, Venier M, Barbieri P, Coceani N, Bussani R, Massiccio M & Spinelli P (2004) In vitro percutaneous absorption of cobalt. Int Arch Occup Environ Health, **77**: 85–89.

Law S, Wertz PW, Swartzendruber DC & Squier CA (1995) Regional variation in content, composition and organization of porcine epithelial barrier lipids revealed by thin-layer chromatography and transmission electron microscopy. Arch Oral Biol, **40**: 1085–1091.

Leveque N, Makki S, Hadgraft J & Humbert P (2004) Comparison of Franz cells and microdialysis for assessing salicylic acid penetration through human skin. Int J Pharm, **269**(2): 323–328.

Levillain F, Charasson V, El Marbouh L, Poey J & Houin G (1998) In vitro study of the percutaneous absorption of four aromatic amines using hairless rat skin. Arzneimittelforschung, **48**(9): 948–951.

Levitt DG (2003) The use of a physiologically based pharmacokinetic model to evaluate deconvolution measurements of systemic absorption. BMC Clin Pharmacol, **19**: 1–29.

Lien EJ & Gao H (1995) QSAR analysis of skin permeability of various drugs in man as compared to in vivo and in vitro studies in rodents. Pharm Res, **12**(4): 583–587.

Lockley DJ, Howes D & Williams FM (2002) Percutaneous penetration and metabolism of 2-ethoxyethanol. Toxicol Appl Pharmacol, **180**(2): 74–82.

Lockley DJ, Howes D & Williams FM (2004) Cutaneous metabolism of glycol ethers. Arch Toxicol, **17**: 1–16.

Loffler H, Dreher F & Maibach HI (2004) Stratum corneum adhesive tape stripping: influence of anatomical site, application pressure, duration and removal. Br J Dermatol, **151**(4): 746–752.

Lotte C, Wester RC, Rougier A & Maibach HI (1993) Racial differences in the in vivo percutaneous absorption of some organic compounds: a comparison between black, Caucasian and Asian subjects. Arch Dermatol Res, **284**: 456–459.

Maas WJM, van de Sandt JJM & Korinth G (2004) Efficiency of microdialysis for the assessment of percutaneous absorption varies between test compounds. In: Brain KR & Walters KA eds. Perspectives in percutaneous penetration. Vol. 9a. Abstracts of presentations at the ninth international perspectives in percutaneous penetration conference held in La Grande Motte, April 2004. Cardiff, STS Publishing, p 98.

Madison KC (2003) Barrier function of the skin: "La raison d'etre" of the epidermis. J Invest Dermatol, **121**(2): 231–241.

Magnusson BM, Anissimov YG, Cross SE & Roberts MS (2004a) Molecular size as the main determinant of solute maximum flux across the skin. J Invest Dermatol, **122**(4): 993–999.

Magnusson BM, Pugh WJ & Roberts MS (2004b) Simple rules defining the potential of compounds for transdermal delivery or toxicity. Pharm Res, **21**(6): 1047–1054.

Maibach H & Patrick E (2001) Dermatotoxicology. In: Hayes WA ed. Principles and methods of toxicology, 4th ed. Philadelphia, PA, Taylor and Francis, pp 1039–1046.

Mancini AJ (2005) Pediatric dermatology. Pediatr Ann, **34**(3): 161–162.

Mao-Qiang M, Elias PM & Feingold KR (1993) Fatty acids are required for epidermal permeability barrier function. J Clin Invest, **92**: 791–798.

Marquart J, Brouwer DH, Gijsbers JHJ, Links IHM, Warren N & van Hemmen JJ (2003) Determinants of dermal exposure relevant for exposure modelling in regulatory risk assessment. Ann Occup Hyg, **47**(8): 599–607.

Martin D, Valdez J, Boren J & Mayersohn M (2004) Dermal absorption of camphor, menthol, and methyl salicylate in humans. J Clin Pharmacol, **44**(10): 1151–1157.

Marzulli FN, Callahan JF & Brown DWC (1965) Chemical structure and skin-penetrating capacity of a short series of organic phosphates and phosphoric acid. J Invest Dermatol, **44**(5): 339–344.

Mathy FX, Lombry C, Verbeeck RK & Preat V (2004) Study of the percutaneous penetration of flurbiprofen by cutaneous and subcutaneous microdialysis after iontophoretic delivery in rat. J Pharm Sci, **94**(1): 144–152.

Mattorano DA, Kupper LL & Nylander-French LA (2004) Estimating dermal exposure to jet fuel (naphthalene) using adhesive tape strip samples. Ann Occup Hyg, **48**(2): 139–146.

McCarley KD & Bunge AL (1998a) Physiologically relevant one-compartment pharmacokinetic models for skin. 1. Development of models. J Pharm Sci, **87**(4): 470–481.

McCarley KD & Bunge AL (1998b) Corrections and additions. Physiologically relevant one-compartment pharmacokinetic models for skin. 1. Development of models. J Pharm Sci, **87**(10): 1264.

McCarley KD & Bunge AL (2000) Physiologically relevant two-compartment models for skin. J Pharm Sci, **89**: 1212–1235.

McCarley KD & Bunge AL (2001) Pharmacokinetic models of dermal absorption. J Pharm Sci, **90**(11): 1699–1719.

McCleverty D, Lyons R & Henry B (2006) Microdialysis sampling and the clinical determination of topical dermal bioequivalence. Int J Pharm, **308**(1–2): 1–7.

McDougal JN & Boeniger MF (2002) Methods for assessing risks of dermal exposures in the workplace. Crit Rev Toxicol, **32**(4): 291–327.

Meuling WJ, Ravensberg LC, Roza L & van Hemmen JJ (2005) Dermal absorption of chlorpyrifos in human volunteers. Int Arch Occup Environ Health, **78**: 44–50.

Michaels AS, Chandrasekaran SK & Shaw JE (1975) Drug permeation through human skin: theory and in vitro experimental measurement. AIChE J, **21**(5): 985–996.

Miselnicky SR, Lichtin JL, Sakr A & Bronaugh RL (1988) The influence of solubility, protein binding, and percutaneous absorption on reservoir formation in skin. J Soc Cosmet Chem, **39**: 167–177.

Monteiro-Riviere NA (2004) Anatomical factors affecting barrier function. In: Zaih H & Maibach HI eds. Dermatotoxicology. Boca Raton, FL, CRC Press, pp 43–70.

Monteiro-Riviere N (2005) Structure and function of skin. In: Riviere JE ed. Dermal absorption models in toxicology and pharmacology. Boca Raton, FL, Taylor & Francis, pp 1–19.

Moody RP (1997) Automated in vitro dermal absorption (AIVDA): A new in vitro method for investigating transdermal flux. Altern Lab Anim, **25**: 347–357.

Moody RP (1998) Bathing water: percutaneous absorption of water contaminants. In: Roberts MS & Walters KA eds. Dermal absorption and toxicity assessment. New York, Marcel Dekker, pp 709–725 (Drugs and the Pharmaceutical Sciences Vol. 91).

Moody RP (2000) Automated in vitro dermal absorption (AIVDA): predicting skin permeation of atrazine with finite and infinite (swimming/bathing) exposure models. Toxicol In Vitro, **14**(5): 467–474.

Moody RP, Franklin CA, Ritter L & Maibach HI (1990) Dermal absorption of the phenoxy herbicides 2,4-D, 2,4-D amine, 2,4-D isooctyl, and 2,4,5-T in rabbits, rats, rhesus monkeys, and humans: a cross species comparison. J Toxicol Environ Health, **29**(3): 237–245.

Moody R, Nadeau B & Chu I (1995) In vivo and in vitro dermal absorption of benzo[*a*]pyrene in rat, guinea pig, human and tissue-cultured skin. J Dermatol Sci, **9**: 48–58.

Moss GP & Cronin MTD (2002) Quantitative structure–permeability relationships for percutaneous absorption: re-analysis of steroid data. Int J Pharm, **238**: 105–109.

Moss T, Howes D & Williams FM (2000) Percutaneous penetration and dermal metabolism of triclosan (2,4,4'-trichloro-2'-hydroxydiphenyl ether). Food Chem Toxicol, **38**(4): 361–370.

Moss GP, Dearden JC, Patel H & Cronin MD (2002) Quantitative structure–permeability relationships (QSPRs) for percutaneous absorption. Toxicol In Vitro, **16**: 299–317.

Mráz J & Nohová H (1992) Percutaneous absorption of *N*,*N*-dimethylformamide in humans. Int Arch Occup Environ Health, **64**: 79–83.

Mueller B, Anissimov YG & Roberts MS (2003) Unexpected clobetasol propionate in human stratum corneum after topical application in vitro. Pharm Res, **20**(11): 1835–1837.

Muller M, Mascher H, Kikuta C, Schafer S, Brunner M, Dorner G & Eichler HG (1997) Diclofenac concentrations in defined tissue layers after topical administration. Clin Pharmacol Ther, **62**(3): 293–299.

Muller RH, Radtke M & Wissing SA (2002) Solid lipid nanoparticles (SLN) and nano-structured lipid carriers (NLC) in cosmetic and dermatological preparations. Adv Drug Deliv Rev, **54**(Suppl. 1): S131–S155.

Nathan D, Sakr A, Lichtin J & Bronaugh R (1990) In vitro skin absorption and metabolism of benzoic acid, *p*-aminobenzoic acid, and benzocaine in the hairless guinea pig. Pharm Res, **7**: 1147–1151.

Ng KME, Chu I, Bronaugh RL, Franklin CA & Somers DA (1991) Percutaneous absorption/metabolism of phenanthrene in the hairless guinea pig: Comparison of in vitro and in vivo results. Fundam Appl Toxicol, **16**: 517–524.

Ng KME, Chu I, Bronaugh RL, Franklin CA & Somers DA (1992) Percutaneous absorption and metabolism of pyrene, benzo[a]pyrene, and di(2-ethylhexyl)phthalate: Comparison of in vitro and in vivo results in the hairless guinea pig. Toxicol Appl Pharmacol, **115**: 216–223.

Nielsen JB (2005) Slightly damaged skin changes the penetration characteristics of four pesticides. In: Proceedings of the second international conference on occupational and environmental exposures of skin to chemicals – 2005, 12–15 June, Stockholm, Sweden. Co-sponsored by the National Institute for Occupational Safety and Health and Karolinska Institutet, Abstract P85, pp 153–154 (http://www.cdc.gov/niosh/topics/skin/OEESC2/authorindex.html).

Nielsen JB & Grandjean P (2004) Criteria for skin notation in different countries. Am J Ind Med, **45**(3): 275–280.

Nielsen JB, Sorensen JA & Nielsen F (2004a) Percutaneous penetration of five pesticides — effects of molecular weight and solubility characteristics. In: Brain KR & Walters KA eds. Perspectives in percutaneous penetration. Vol. 9a. Abstracts of presentations at the ninth international perspectives in percutaneous penetration conference held in La Grande Motte, April 2004. Cardiff, STS Publishing, p 103.

Nielsen JB, Nielsen F & Sorensen JA (2004b) In vitro percutaneous penetration of five pesticides — effects of molecular weight and solubility characteristics. Ann Occup Hyg, **48**(8): 697–705.

Nielsen JB, Sartorelli P & Grandjean P (2004c) A semi-quantitative approach to skin notation. In: Brain KR & Walters KA eds. Perspectives in percutaneous penetration. Vol. 9a. Abstracts of presentations at the ninth international perspectives in percutaneous penetration conference held in La Grande Motte, April 2004. Cardiff, STS Publishing, p 104.

Nitsche JM, Wang TF & Kasting GB (2006) A two-phase analysis of solute partitioning into the stratum corneum. J Pharm Sci, **95**(3): 649–666.

Nohynek GJ, Meuling WJ, Vaes WH, Lawrence RS, Shapiro S, Schulte S, Steiling W, Bausch J, Gerber E, Sasa H & Nau H (2006) Repeated topical treatment, in contrast to single oral doses, with vitamin A–containing preparations does not affect plasma concentrations of retinol, retinyl esters or retinoic acids in female subjects of child-bearing age. Toxicol Lett, **163**(1): 65–76.

Nomiyama T, Omae K, Ishizuka C, Yamauchi T, Kawasumi Y, Yamada K, Endoh H & Sakurai H (2000) Dermal absorption of *N,N*-dimethylacetamide in human volunteers. Int Arch Occup Environ Health, **73**(2): 121–126.

Nomiyama T, Nakashima H, Chen LL, Tanaka S, Miyauchi H, Yamauchi T, Sakurai H & Omae K (2001) *N,N*-Dimethylformamide: significance of dermal absorption and adjustment method for urinary *N*-methylformamide concentration as a biological exposure item. Int Arch Occup Environ Health, **74**(3): 224–228.

O'Connor J & Cage S (2004) In vitro skin absorption — can it be used in isolation for risk assessment purposes? In: Brain KR & Walters KA eds. Perspectives in percutaneous penetration. Vol. 9a. Abstracts of presentations at the ninth international perspectives in percutaneous penetration conference held in La Grande Motte, April 2004. Cardiff, STS Publishing, p 92.

O'Connor J, Cage S & Fong L (2004) In vitro skin absorption — can it be used in isolation for risk assessment purposes? Poster at the ninth international perspectives in percutaneous penetration conference held in La Grande Motte, April 2004.

OECD (2000) Test Guidelines Programme. Percutaneous absorption testing: is there a way to consensus? Paris, Organisation for Economic Co-operation and Development, pp 1–42 (ENV/JM/TG(2000)5) [cited in EC, 2004].

OECD (2004a) Guidance document for the conduct of skin absorption studies. Paris, Organisation for Economic Co-operation and Development, Environment Directorate, March, pp 1–31 (OECD Environmental Health and Safety Publications Series on Testing and Assessment No. 28; ENV/JM/MONO(2004)2; http://appli1.oecd.org/olis/2004doc.nsf/linkto/env-jm-mono(2004)2).

OECD (2004b) OECD guideline for the testing of chemicals. Skin absorption: in vivo method. 427. Adopted: 13 April 2004. Paris, Organisation for Economic Co-operation and Development, pp 1–8.

OECD (2004c) OECD guideline for the testing of chemicals. Skin absorption: in vitro method. 428. Adopted: 13 April 2004. Paris, Organisation for Economic Co-operation and Development, pp 1–8.

OECD (2004d) OECD guideline for the testing of chemicals. Partition coefficient (*n*-octanol/water), high performance liquid chromatography (HPLC) method. 117. Adopted: 13 April 2004. Paris, Organisation for Economic Co-operation and Development.

O'Neill D & Fitzpatrick D (2004) Determination using HPLC of partition and distribution coefficients, for use in transdermal modelling. In: Brain KR & Walters KA eds. Perspectives in percutaneous penetration. Vol. 9a. Abstracts of presentations at the ninth international perspectives in percutaneous penetration conference held in La Grande Motte, April 2004. Cardiff, STS Publishing, p 93.

Oppl R, Kalberlah F, Evans PG & van Hemmen JJ (2003) A toolkit for dermal risk assessment and management: an overview. Ann Occup Hyg, **47**(8): 629–640.

Palenske J & Morhenn VB (1999) Changes in the skin's capacitance after damage to the stratum corneum in humans. J Cutan Med Surg, **3**(3): 127–131.

Pannatier A, Jenner P, Testa B & Etter JC (1978) The skin as a drug-metabolizing organ. Drug Metab Rev, **8**(2): 319–343.

Patel H & Cronin M (2001) Determination of the optimal physico-chemical parameters to use in a QSAR-approach to predict skin permeation rate. Final report. European Chemical Industry Council Long-range Research Initiative, June, 109 pp (CEFIC-LRI Project No. NMALRI-A2.2UNJM-0007, http://www.staff.livjm.ac.uk/phamcron/qsar/CEFIC/final%20report.pdf).

Patel H, ten Berge W & Cronin MT (2002) Quantitative structure–activity relationships (QSARs) for the prediction of skin permeation of exogenous chemicals. Chemosphere, **48**: 603–613.

Pendlington RU, Williams DL, Naik JT & Sharma RK (1994) Distribution of xenobotic metabolising enzymes in skin. Toxicol In Vitro, **8**: 525–527.

Pendlington RU, Sanders DJ, Bourner CB, Saunders DR & Pease CK (2004) Development of a repeat dose in vitro skin penetration model. In: Brain KR & Walters KA eds. Perspectives in percutaneous penetration. Vol. 9a. Abstracts of presentations at the ninth international perspectives in percutaneous penetration conference held in La Grande Motte, April 2004. Cardiff, STS Publishing, p 79.

Pershing LK, Bakhtian S, Poncelet CE, Corlett JL & Shah VP (2002a) Comparison of skin stripping, in vitro release, and skin blanching response methods to measure dose response and similarity of triamcinolone acetonide cream strengths from two manufactured sources. J Pharm Sci, **91**(5): 1312–1323.

Pershing LK, Corlett JL & Nelson JL (2002b) Comparison of dermatopharmacokinetic vs. clinical efficacy methods for bioequivalence assessment of miconazole nitrate vaginal cream, 2% in humans. Pharm Res, **19**: 270–277.

Pershing LK, Nelson JL, Corlett JL, Shrivastava SP, Hare DB & Shah VP (2003) Assessment of dermatopharmacokinetic approach in the bioequivalence determination of topical tretinoin gel products. J Am Acad Dermatol, **48**(5): 740–751.

Pilgram GS, Engelsma-van Pelt AM, Bouwstra JA & Koerten HK (1999) Electron diffraction provides new information on human stratum corneum lipid organization studied in relation to depth and temperature. J Invest Dermatol, **113**(3): 403–409.

Piotrowski JK (1971) Evaluation of exposure to phenol: absorption of phenol vapor in the lungs and through the skin and excretion of phenol in urine. Br J Ind Med, **28**(2): 172–178.

Pirot F, Berardesca E, Kalia YN, Singh M, Maibach HI & Guy RH (1998) Stratum corneum thickness and apparent water diffusivity: facile and noninvasive quantitation in vivo. Pharm Res, **15**(3): 492–494.

Poda GI, Landsittel DP, Brumbaugh K, Sharp DS, Frasch HF & Demchuk E (2001) Random sampling or "random" model in skin flux measurements? [Commentary on "Investigation of the mechanisms of flux across human skin in vitro by quantitative structure–permeability relationship", Eur J Pharm Sci 1999 Mar;7(4):325–330.] Eur J Pharm Sci, **14**(3): 197–200.

Ponec M, Gibbs S, Pilgram G, Boelsma E, Koerten H, Bouwstra J & Mommaas M (2001) Barrier function in reconstructed epidermis and its resemblance to native human skin. Skin Pharmacol Appl Skin Physiol, **14**(Suppl. 1): 63–71.

Ponec M, Weerheim A, Lankhorst P & Wertz P (2003) New acylceramide in native and reconstructed epidermis. J Invest Dermatol, **120**(4): 581–588.

Potts RO & Guy RH (1992) Predicting skin permeability. Pharm Res, **9**(5): 663–669.

Potts RO & Guy RH (1995) A predictive algorithm for skin permeability: the effects of molecular size and hydrogen bond activity. Pharm Res, **12**(11): 1628–1633.

Pugh W & Hadgraft J (1994) Ab initio prediction of human skin permeability coefficients. Int J Pharm, **103**: 163–178.

Ramsey JD, Woollen BH, Auton TR, Batten PL & Leeser JE (1992) Pharmacokinetics of fluazifop-butyl in human volunteers. II: Dermal dosing. Hum Exp Toxicol, **11**(4): 247–254.

Ramsey JD, Woollen BH, Auton TR & Scott RC (1994) The predictive accuracy of in vitro measurements for the dermal absorption of a lipophilic penetrant (fluazifop-butyl) through rat and human skin. Fundam Appl Toxicol, **23**: 230–236.

Rawlings AV & Matts PJ (2005) Stratum corneum moisturization at the molecular level: an update in relation to the dry skin cycle. J Invest Dermatol, **124**(6): 1099–1110.

Raykar PV, Fung MC & Anderson BD (1988) The role of protein and lipid domains in the uptake of solutes by human stratum corneum. Pharm Res, **5**(3): 140–150.

Reddy MB & Bunge AL (2002) Dermal absorption of chemical residues: Data analysis. In: Krüse J, Verhaar H & de Raat WK eds. The practical applicability of toxicokinetic models in the risk assessment of chemicals. Dordrecht, Kluwer Academic Publishers, pp 44–78.

Reddy MB, McCarley KD & Bunge AL (1998) Physiologically relevant one-compartment pharmacokinetic models for skin. 2. Comparison of models when combined with a systemic pharmacokinetic model. J Pharm Sci, **87**: 482–490.

Reddy MB, Stinchcomb AL, Guy RH & Bunge AL (2002) Determining dermal absorption parameters in vivo from tape strip data. Pharm Res, **19**(3): 292–298.

Ridout G & Guy RH (1988) Structure–penetration relationships in percutaneous absorption. ACS Symp Ser, **371**: 112–123.

Ridout G, Houk J, Guy R, Santus GC, Hadgraft J & Hall LL (1992) An evaluation of structure–penetration relationships in percutaneous absorption. Farmaco (Pavia), **47**(6): 869–892.

Rigg PC & Barry BW (1990) Shed snake skin and hairless mouse skin as model membranes for human skin during permeation studies. J Invest Dermatol, **94**(2): 235–240.

Riihimaki V & Pfaffli P (1978) Percutaneous absorption of solvent vapors in man. Scand J Work Environ Health, **4**(1): 73–85.

Roberts MS & Anissimov Y (2005) Mathematical models in percutaneous absorption. In: Bronaugh RL & Maibach HI eds. Percutaneous absorption: drugs, cosmetics, mechanisms, methodology, 4th ed. Boca Raton, FL, Taylor & Francis, pp 1–44 (Drugs and the Pharmaceutical Sciences Vol. 155).

Roberts MS & Horlock E (1978) Effect of repeated application of salicylic acid to the skin on its percutaneous absorption. J Pharm Sci, **67**: 1685–1687.

Roberts MS & Walker M (1993) Water — the most natural penetration enhancer. In: Walters KA & Hadgraft J eds. Pharmaceutical skin penetration enhancement. New York, Marcel Dekker, pp 1–30.

Roberts MS & Walters KA (1998) The relationship between structure and barrier function of skin. In: Roberts MS & Walters KA eds. Dermal absorption and toxicity assessment. New York, Marcel Dekker, pp 1–42.

Roberts MS, Anderson RA & Swarbrick J (1977) Permeability of human epidermis to phenolic compounds. J Pharm Pharmacol, **29**: 677–683.

Roberts MS, Favretto WA, Meyer A, Reckmann M & Wongseelashote T (1982) Topical bioavailability of methyl salicylate. Aust N Z J Med, **12**: 303–305.

Roberts MS, Pugh WJ & Hadgraft J (1996) Epidermal permeability–penetrant structure relationships: 2. The effect of H-bonding groups in penetrants on their diffusion through stratum corneum. Int J Pharm, **132**: 23–33.

Roberts MS, Lai PM & Anissimov YG (1998) Epidermal iontophoresis: 1. Development of the ionic mobility-pore model. Pharm Res, **15**: 1569–1578.

Roberts MS, Anissimov YG & Gonsalvez RA (1999) Mathematical models in percutaneous absorption. In: Bronaugh RL & Maibach HI eds. Percutaneous absorption: drugs–cosmetics–mechanisms–methodology, 3rd ed. New York, Marcel Dekker, pp 3–55 (Drugs and the Pharmaceutical Sciences Vol. 97).

Roberts MS, Cross SE & Pellett MA (2002) Skin transport. In Walters KA ed. Dermatological and transdermal formulations. New York, Marcel Dekker, pp 89–195 (Drugs and the Pharmaceutical Sciences Vol. 119).

Roberts MS, Cross SE & Anissmov YG (2004) Factors affecting the formation of a skin reservoir for topically applied solutes. Skin Pharmacol Physiol, **17**(1): 3–16.

Romani N, Holzmann S, Tripp CH, Koch F & Stoitzner P (2003) Langerhans cells — dendritic cells of the epidermis. Acta Pathol Microbiol Immunol Scand, **111**(7–8): 725–740.

Romonchuk WJ & Bunge AL (2003) Absorption of 4-cyanophenol from powder and saturated aqueous solution into silicone rubber membranes and human skin. American Association of Pharmaceutical Scientists Annual Meeting and Exposition, Salt Lake City, UT, 26–30 October 2003.

Romonchuk WJ & Bunge AL (2004) Temperature variations in diffusion cell systems. In: Brain KR & Walters KA eds. Perspectives in percutaneous penetration. Vol. 9a. Abstracts of presentations at the ninth international perspectives in percutaneous penetration conference held in La Grande Motte, April 2004. Cardiff, STS Publishing, p 86.

Roper CS, Crow LF & Madden S (2004) Should we use a barrier integrity test for skin barrier function of human skin in skin penetration studies? In: Brain KR & Walters KA eds. Perspectives in percutaneous penetration. Vol. 9a. Abstracts of presentations at the ninth international perspectives in percutaneous penetration conference held in La Grande Motte, April 2004. Cardiff, STS Publishing, p 69.

Roskos KV, Maibach HI & Guy RH (1989) The effect of aging on percutaneous absorption in man. J Pharmacokinet Biopharm, **17**(6): 617–630.

Ross JH, Driver JH, Harris SA & Maibach HI (2005) Dermal absorption of 2,4-D: a review of species differences. Regul Toxicol Pharmacol, **41**(1): 82–91.

Rougier A, Lotte C & Maibach HI (1987) In vivo percutaneous penetration of some organic compounds related to anatomic site in humans: Predictive assessment by the stripping method. J Pharm Sci, **76**: 451–454.

Rougier A, Dupuis D, Lotte C & Maibach HI (1999) Stripping method for measuring percutaneous absorption in vivo. In: Bronaugh RL & Maibach HI eds. Percutaneous absorption: drugs–cosmetics–mechanisms–methodology, 3rd ed. New York, Marcel Dekker, pp 375–393 (Drugs and the Pharmaceutical Sciences Vol. 97).

Roy TA, Krueger AJ, Mackerer CR, Neil W, Arroyo AM & Yang JJ (1998) SAR models for estimating the percutaneous absorption of polynuclear aromatic hydrocarbons. SAR QSAR Environ Res, **9**: 171–185.

Rushmer RF, Buettner KJK, Short JM & Odland GF (1966) The skin. Science, **154**(3747): 343–348.

Saiyasombati P & Kasting GB (2003) Disposition of benzyl alcohol after topical application to human skin in vitro. J Pharm Sci, **92**(10): 2128–2139 [Erratum in: J Pharm Sci, 2003, **92**(12): 2534].

Saleh MA, Ahmed AE, Kamel A & Dary C (1997) Determination of the distribution of malathion in rats following various routes of administration by whole-body electronic autoradiography. Toxicol Ind Health, **13**(6): 751–758.

Santos Maia C, Mehnert W, Schaller M, Korting HC, Gysler A, Haberland A & Schafer-Korting M (2002) Drug targeting by solid lipid nanoparticles for dermal use. J Drug Target, **10**(6): 489–495.

Sartorelli P (2002) Dermal exposure assessment in occupational medicine. Occup Med, **52**(3): 151–156.

Sartorelli P, Andersen HR, Angerer J, Corish J, Drexler H, Göen T, Griffin P, Hotchkiss SAM, Larese F, Montomoli L, Perkins J, Schmelz M, van de Sandt J & Williams F (2000) Percutaneous penetration studies for risk assessment. Environ Toxicol Pharmacol, **8**(2): 133–152.

Sartorelli P, Montomoli L, Cioni F & Sisinni AG (2004) In vitro percutaneous absorption of metals. In: Brain KR & Walters KA eds. Perspectives in percutaneous penetration. Vol. 9a. Abstracts of presentations at the ninth international perspectives in percutaneous penetration conference held in La Grande Motte, April 2004. Cardiff, STS Publishing, p 102.

Saunders M & Pugh W (2002) Use of ethanol in receptor phase — a lucky escape? In: Brain KR & Walters KA eds. Perspectives in percutaneous penetration. Vol 8a. Abstracts of presentations at the eighth international perspectives in percutaneous penetration conference held in Antibes-Juan-les-Prins, April 2002. Cardiff, STS Publishing, p 21.

SCCNFP (2003a) Notes of guidance for testing of cosmetic ingredients for their safety evaluation, 5th revision, adopted by the SCCNFP during 25th plenary meeting of 20

October 2003. Scientific Committee on Cosmetic Products and Non-Food Products Intended for Consumers, pp 1–102 (SCCNFP/069003, Final).

SCCNFP (2003b) Basic criteria for the in vitro assessment of dermal absorption of cosmetic ingredients, updated October 2003, adopted by the SCCNFP during the 25th plenary meeting of 20 October 2003. Scientific Committee on Cosmetic Products and Non-Food Products Intended for Consumers, pp 1–9 (SCCNFP/0750/03).

SCENIHR (2005) Scientific Committee on Emerging and Newly Identified Health Risks (SCENIHR) opinion on the appropriateness of existing methodologies to assess the potential risks associated with engineered and adventitious products of nanotechnologies. Adopted by the SCENIHR during the 7th plenary meeting of 28–29 September 2005 (SCENIHR 002/005; http://europa.eu.int/comm/health/ph_risk/committees/04_scenihr/docs/scenihr_o_003.pdf).

Schaefer H & Redelmeier TE (1996) Skin barrier: principles of percutaneous absorption. Basel, Schweiz, S. Karger AG, pp 1–310.

Schaefer H & Stuttgen G (1976) Absolute concentrations of an antimycotic agent, econazole, in the human skin after local application. Arzneimittelforschung, **26**(3): 432–435.

Schaefer H, Zesch A & Stuttgen G (1977) Penetration, permeation, and absorption of triamcinolone acetonide in normal and psoriatic skin. Arch Dermatol Res, **258**(3): 241–249.

Schaefer H, Stuttgen G, Zesch A, Schalla W & Gazith J (1978) Quantitative determination of percutaneous absorption of radiolabeled drugs in vitro and in vivo by human skin. Curr Probl Dermatol, **7**: 80–94.

Schäfer P, Bewick-Sonntag C, Capri MG & Berardesca E (2002) Physiological changes in skin barrier function in relation to occlusion level, exposure time and climatic conditions. Skin Pharmacol Appl Skin Physiol, **15**: 7–19.

Scheuplein RJ (1967) Mechanism of percutaneous absorption. II. Transient diffusion and the relative importance of barrier routes of skin penetration. J Invest Dermatol, **48**: 79.

Scheuplein RJ & Blank IH (1971) Permeability of the skin. Physiol Rev, **51**(4): 702–747.

Scheuplein RJ & Blank IH (1973) Mechanism of percutaneous absorption. IV. Penetration of nonelectrolytes (alcohols) from solutions and from pure liquids. J Invest Dermatol, **60**(5): 286–296.

Scheuplein RJ & Ross EW (1974) Mechanism of percutaneous absorption. V Percutaneous absorption of solvent deposited solids. J Invest Dermatol, **62**: 353–360.

Scheuplein RJ, Blank IH, Brauner GJ & MacFarlane DJ (1969) Percutaneous absorption of steroids. J Invest Dermatol, **52**: 63–70.

Schneider T, Vermeulen R, Brouwer DH, Cherrie JW, Kromhout H & Fogh CL (1999) Conceptual model for assessment of dermal exposure. Occup Environ Med, **56**: 765–773.

Schnetz E & Fartasch M (2001) Microdialysis for the evaluation of penetration through the human skin barrier — a promising tool for future research? Eur J Pharm Sci, **12**(3): 165–174.

Scholer N, Zimmermann E, Katzfey U, Hahn H, Muller RH & Liesenfeld O (2000) Effect of solid lipid nanoparticles (SLN) on cytokine production and the viability of murine peritoneal macrophages. J Microencapsul, **17**(5): 639–650.

Scott RC & Ramsey JD (1987) Comparison of the in vivo and in vitro percutaneous absorption of a lipophilic molecule (cypermethrin, a pyrethroid insecticide). J Invest Dermatol, **89**: 142–146.

Scott RC, Walker M & Dugart PH (1986) A comparison of the in vitro permeability properties of human and some laboratory animal skins. Int J Cosmet Sci, **8**: 189–194.

Scott RC, Guy RH & Hadgraft J eds (1990) Prediction of percutaneous penetration. London, IBC Technical Services Ltd (ISBN 1 85271 117 5).

Scott RC, Corrigan MA, Smith F & Mason H (1991a) The influence of skin structure on permeability: an intersite and interspecies comparison with hydrophilic penetrants. J Invest Dermatol, **96**: 921–925.

Scott RC, Guy RH, Hadgraft J & Bodde HE eds (1991b) Prediction of percutaneous penetration. Vol. 2. London, IBC Technical Services Ltd (ISBN 1 85271 187 6).

Scott RC, Batten PL, Clowes HM, Jones BK & Ramsey JD (1992) Further validation of an in vitro method to reduce the need for in vivo studies for measuring the absorption of chemicals through rat skin. Fundam Appl Toxicol, **19**: 484–492.

Semple S (2004) Dermal exposure to chemicals in the workplace: just how important is skin absorption? Occup Environ Med, **61**(4): 376–382.

Shah JC (1993) Analysis of permeation data: evaluation of the lag time method. Int J Pharm, **90**: 161–169.

Shah VP, Flynn GL, Yacobi A, Maibach HI, Bon C, Fleischer NM, Franz TJ, Kaplan SA, Kawamoto J, Lesko LJ, Marty JP, Pershing LK, Schaefer H, Sequeira JA, Shrivastava SP, Wilkin J & Williams RL (1998) Bioequivalence of topical dermatological dosage forms — methods of evaluation of bioequivalence. Pharm Res, **15**(2): 167–171.

Shvedova AA, Castranova V, Kisin ER, Schwegler-Berry D, Murray AR, Gandelsman VZ, Maynard A & Baron P (2003) Exposure to carbon nanotube material: assessment of nanotube cytotoxicity using human keratinocyte cells. J Toxicol Environ Health A, **66**(20): 1909–1926.

Siddiqui O, Roberts MS & Polack AE (1989) Percutaneous absorption of steroids: relative contributions of epidermal penetration and dermal clearance. J Pharmacokinet Biopharm, **17**(4): 405–424.

Simonsen L, Petersen MB & Groth L (2002) In vivo skin penetration of salicylic compounds in hairless rats. Eur J Pharm Sci, **17**(1–2): 95–104.

Singh P & Roberts MS (1994) Effects of vasoconstriction on dermal pharmacokinetics and local tissue distribution of compounds. J Pharm Sci, **83**(6): 783–791.

Singh S & Singh J (1993) Transdermal drug delivery by passive diffusion and iontophoresis: a review. Med Res Rev, **13**(5): 569–621.

Skelly JP, Shan VP, Guy RH, Wester RC, Flynn G & Yacobi A (1987) FDA and AAPS report of the workshop on principles and practices of in vitro percutaneous penetration studies: relevance to bioavailability and bioequivalence. Pharm Res, **4**(3): 265–267.

Southwell JD, Barry BW & Woodford R (1984) Variations in permeability of human skin within and between specimens. Int J Pharm, **18**: 299–309.

Souto EB, Wissing SA, Barbosa CM & Muller RH (2004) Comparative study between the viscoelastic behavior of different lipid nanoparticle formulations. J Cosmet Sci, **55**(5): 463–471.

Soyei S & Williams F (2004) A database of percutaneous absorption, distribution and physicochemical parameters. In: Brain KR & Walters KA eds. Perspectives in percutaneous penetration. Vol. 9a. Abstracts of presentations at the ninth international perspectives in percutaneous penetration conference held in La Grande Motte, April 2004. Cardiff, STS Publishing, p 84.

Steiling W, Kreutz J & Hofer H (2001) Percutaneous penetration/dermal absorption of hair dyes in vitro. Toxicol In Vitro, **15**: 565–570.

Stempfer B & Bunge AL (2004) How much chemical in the skin will evaporate? In: Brain KR & Walters KA eds. Perspectives in percutaneous penetration. Vol. 9a. Abstracts of presentations at the ninth international perspectives in percutaneous penetration conference held in La Grande Motte, April 2004. Cardiff, STS Publishing, p 88.

Surber C, Schwarb FP & Smith EW (1999) Tape-stripping technique. In: Bronaugh RL & Maibach HI eds. Percutaneous absorption: drugs–cosmetics–mechanisms–methodology, 3rd ed. New York, Marcel Dekker, pp 395–409 (Drugs and the Pharmaceutical Sciences Vol. 97).

Suskind RR (1977) Environment and skin. Environ Health Perspect, **20**: 27–37.

Tan MH, Commens CA, Burnett L & Snitch PJ (1996) A pilot study on the percutaneous absorption of microfine titanium dioxide from sunscreens. Australas J Dermatol, **37**: 185–187.

Tanojo H, Bouwstra JA, Junginger HE & Boddé HE (1997) In vitro human skin barrier modulation by fatty acids: skin permeation and thermal analysis studies. Pharm Res, **14**(1): 42–49.

Tauber U & Matthes H (1992) Percutaneous absorption of methylprednisolone aceponate after single and multiple dermal application as ointment in male volunteers. Arzneimittelforschung, **42**(9): 1122–1124.

ten Berge WF (2005) Modelling dermal exposure and absorption through the skin. 11 pp (http://home.planet.nl/~wtberge/skinperm.html).

Tezel A, Sens A & Mitragotri S (2003) Description of transdermal transport of hydrophilic solutes during low-frequency sonophoresis based on a modified porous pathway model. J Pharm Sci, **92**(2): 381–393.

Thongsinthusak TH, Ross JH, Saiz SG & Krieger RI (1999) Estimation of dermal absorption using the exponential saturation model. Regul Toxicol Pharmacol, **29**: 37–43.

Tinkle SS, Antonini JM, Rich BA, Roberts JR, Salmen R, Depree K & Adkins EJ (2003) Particle penetration of the skin as a route of exposure in chronic beryllium disease. Environ Health Perspect, **119**(9): 1202–1208.

Trebilcock KL, Heylings JR & Wilks MF (1994) In vitro tape stripping as a model for in vivo skin stripping. Toxicol In Vitro, **8**: 665–667.

Tsai JC, Sheu HM, Hung PL & Cheng CL (2001) Effect of barrier disruption by acetone treatment on the permeability of compounds with various lipophilicities: implications for the permeability of compromised skin. J Pharm Sci, **90**(9): 1242–1254.

Tsai JC, Shen LC, Sheu HM & Lu CC (2003) Tape stripping and sodium dodecyl sulfate treatment increase the molecular weight cutoff of polyethylene glycol penetration across murine skin. Arch Dermatol Res, **295**: 169–174.

Tsuji JS, Maynard AD, Howard PC, James JT, Lam CW, Warheit DB & Santamaria AB (2006) Research strategies for safety evaluation of nanomaterials, Part IV: Risk assessment of nanoparticles. Toxicol Sci, **89**(1): 42–50.

Turner P, Saeed B & Kelsey MC (2004) Dermal absorption of isopropyl alcohol from a commercial hand rub: implications for its use in hand decontamination. J Hosp Infect, **56**(4): 287–290.

Ursin C, Hansen CM, Van Dyk JW, Jensen PO, Christensen IJ & Ebbehoej J (1995) Permeability of commercial solvents through living human skin. Am Ind Hyg Assoc J, **56**: 651–660.

USEPA (1992) Dermal exposure assessment: principles and applications. Interim report. Washington, DC, United States Environmental Protection Agency, Office of Health and Environmental Assessment pp 1–389 (EPA/600/8-91/011B; http://www.epa.gov/nceawww1/pdfs/derexp.pdf).

USEPA (1998) Health effects test guidelines. OPPTS 870.7600. Dermal penetration. Washington, DC, United States Environmental Protection Agency, Office of Prevention, Pesticides and Toxic Substances, pp 1–12 (http://www.epa.gov/opptsfrs/publications/OPPTS_Harmonized/870_Health_Effects_Test_Guidelines/Series/870-7600.pdf).

USEPA (1999) Proposed test rule for in vitro dermal absorption rate testing of certain chemicals of interest to Occupational Safety and Health Administration; Proposed rule. Fed Regist, **64**(110): 31073–31090.

USEPA (2004a) In vitro dermal absorption rate testing of certain chemicals of interest to the Occupational Safety and Health Administration; Final rule. Fed Regist, **69**(80): 22402–22441.

USEPA (2004b) Risk assessment guidance for Superfund, Vol. I: Human health evaluation manual (part E, supplemental guidance for dermal risk assessment). Final. Washington, DC, United States Environmental Protection Agency, Office of Superfund Remediation and Technology Innovation, pp 1–156 (EPA540/R/99/005; http://www.epa.gov/oswer/riskassessment/ragse/pdf/introduction.pdf).

USFDA (1998) Guidance for industry: topical dermatological drug product NDAs and ANDAs — in vivo bioavailability, bioequivalence, in vitro release, and associated studies. Draft guidance, June 1998. Rockville, MD, United States Department of Health and Human Services, Food and Drug Administration, Center for Drug Evaluation and Research.

USFDA (2001) CDER Advisory Committee for Pharmaceutical Science Committee Meeting, 28–29 November 2001. Rockville, MD, United States Department of Health and Human Services, Food and Drug Administration (http://www.fda.gov/ohrms/dockets/).

Valiveti S, Paudel KS, Hammell DC, Hamad MO, Chen J, Crooks PA & Stinchcomb AL (2005) In vitro/in vivo correlation of transdermal naltrexone prodrugs in hairless guinea pigs. Pharm Res, **22**(6): 981–989.

Vanakoski J, Seppälä T, Sievi E & Lunell E (1996) Exposure to high ambient temperature increases absorption and plasma concentrations of transdermal nicotine. Clin Pharmacol Ther, **60**(3). 308–315.

van der Molen RG, Spies F, van't Noordende JM, Boelsma E, Mommaas AM & Koerten HK (1997) Tape stripping of human stratum corneum yields cell layers that originate from various depths because of furrows in the skin. Arch Dermatol Res, **289**(9): 514–518.

van de Sandt JJM (2004) In vitro predictions of skin absorption: robustness and critical factors. In: Brain KR & Walters KA eds. Perspectives in percutaneous penetration. Vol. 9a. Abstracts of presentations at the ninth international perspectives in percutaneous penetration conference held in La Grande Motte, April 2004. Cardiff, STS Publishing, p 7.

van de Sandt JJM, Rutten AAJJL & van Ommen B (1993) Species specific cutaneous biotransformation of the pesticide propoxur during percutaneous absorption in vitro. Toxicol Appl Pharmacol, **123**: 144–150.

van de Sandt JJM, Meuling WJA, Elliott GR, Cnubben NHP & Hakkert B (2000) Comparative in vitro–in vivo percutaneous absorption of the pesticide propoxur. Toxicol Sci, **58**: 15–22.

van de Sandt JJM, van Burgsteden JA, Carmichael PL, Dick I, Kenyon S, Korinth G, Larese F, Limasset JC, Maas WJM, Montomoli L, Nielsen JB, Payan J-P, Robinson E, Sartorelli P, Schaller KH, Wilkinson SC & Williams FM (2004) In vitro predictions of skin absorption of caffeine, testosterone, and benzoic acid: a multi-centre comparison study. Regul Toxicol Pharmacol, **39**: 271–281.

van Hemmen JJ (2004) Dermal exposure to chemicals. Ann Occup Hyg, **48**(3): 183–185.

van Hemmen JJ, Auffarth J, Evans PG, Rajan-Sithamparanadarajah B, Marquart H & Oppl R (2003) RISKOFDERM: risk assessment of occupational dermal exposure to chemicals. An introduction to a series of papers on the development of a toolkit. Ann Occup Hyg, **47**(8): 595–598.

van Ravenzwaay B & Leibold E (2004) A comparison between in vitro rat and human and in vivo rat skin absorption studies. Hum Exp Toxicol, **23**(9): 421–430.

van Rooij JGM, Vinke E, de Lange J, Bruijnzeel PLB, Bodelier-Bade MM, Noordhoek J & Jongeneelen FJ (1995) Dermal absorption of polycyclic aromatic hydrocarbons in the blood-perfused pig ear. J Appl Toxicol, **15**(3): 193–200.

Vecchia BE & Bunge AL (2003a) Skin absorption databases and predictive equations. In: Guy R & Hadgraft J eds. Transdermal drug delivery, 2nd ed. New York, Marcel Dekker, pp 57–141 (Drugs and the Pharmaceutical Sciences Vol. 123).

Vecchia BE & Bunge AL (2003b) Evaluating the transdermal permeability of chemicals. In: Guy R & Hadgraft J eds. Transdermal drug delivery, 2nd ed. New York, Marcel Dekker, pp 25–55 (Drugs and the Pharmaceutical Sciences Vol. 123).

Vecchia BE & Bunge AL (2003c) Partitioning of chemicals into skin: Results and predictions. In: Guy R & Hadgraft J eds. Transdermal drug delivery, 2nd ed. New York, Marcel Dekker, pp 143–198 (Drugs and the Pharmaceutical Sciences Vol. 123).

Vecchia BE & Bunge AL (2005) Animal models: a comparison of permeability coefficients for excised skin from humans and animals. In: Riviere JE ed. Dermal absorption models in toxicology and pharmacology. Boca Raton, FL, Taylor & Francis, pp 303–365.

Venier M, Larese F, Adami G & Maina G (2004) In vitro percutaneous absorption of metal powders. In: Brain KR & Walters KA eds. Perspectives in percutaneous penetration. Abstracts of presentations at the ninth international perspectives in percutaneous penetration conference held in La Grande Motte, April 2004. Cardiff, STS Publishing, p 101.

Vickers CF (1972) Stratum corneum reservoir for drugs. Adv Biol Skin, **12**: 177–189.

Wagner H, Kostka KH, Lehr CM & Schaefer UF (2001) Interrelation of permeation and penetration parameters obtained from in vitro experiments with human skin and skin equivalents. J Control Release, **75**(3): 283–295.

Walker JD, Whittaker C & McDougal JN (1996) Role of the TSCA Interagency Testing Committee in meeting the US government's data needs: Designating chemicals for percutaneous absorption testing. In: Marzulli FN & Maibach HI eds. Dermatotoxicology, 5th ed. Washington, DC, Hemisphere Publishing Corporation, pp 371–381.

Walker JD, Rodford R & Patlewicz G (2003) Quantitative structure–activity relationships for predicting percutaneous absorption rates. Environ Toxicol Chem, **22**(8): 1870–1884.

Walters KA & Brain KR (2000) Skin permeation predictions and databases — what are their limitations. In: Perspectives in percutaneous penetration. Vol. 7a. Abstracts of presentations at the seventh international perspectives in percutaneous penetration conference held in La Grande Motte. Cardiff, STS Publishing, p 15 [cited in Moss et al., 2002].

Walters KA & Roberts MS (1993) Veterinary applications of skin penetration enhancers. In: Walters KA & Hadgraft J eds. Pharmaceutical skin penetration enhancement. New York, Marcel Dekker, pp 345–364 (Drugs and the Pharmaceutical Sciences Vol. 59).

Walters KA & Roberts MS (2002) The structure and function of skin. In: Walters KA ed. Dermatological and transdermal formulations. New York, Marcel Dekker, pp 1–39 (Drugs and the Pharmaceutical Sciences Vol. 119).

Walters KA, Gettings SD & Roberts MS (1999) Percutaneous absorption of sunscreens. In: Bronaugh RL & Maibach HI eds. Percutaneous absorption: drugs–cosmetics–mechanisms–methodology, 3rd ed. New York, Marcel Dekker, pp 861–877 (Drugs and the Pharmaceutical Sciences Vol. 97).

Wang TF, Kasting GB & Nitsche JM (2006) A multiphase microscopic diffusion model for stratum corneum permeability. I. Formulation, solution, and illustrative results for representative compounds. J Pharm Sci, **95**(3): 620–648.

Warner RR, Stone KJ & Boissy YL (2003) Hydration disrupts human stratum corneum ultrastructure. J Invest Dermatol, **120**(2): 275–284.

Weigmann H, Lademann J, Meffert H, Schaefer H & Sterry W (1999) Determination of the horny layer profile by tape stripping in combination with optical spectroscopy in the visible range as a prerequisite to quantify percutaneous absorption. Skin Pharmacol Appl Skin Physiol, **12**(1–2): 34–45.

Weigmann HJ, Lademann J, Schanzer S, Lindemann U, von Pelchrzim R, Schaefer H, Sterry W & Shah V (2001) Correlation of the local distribution of topically applied substances inside the stratum corneum determined by tape-stripping to differences in bioavailability. Skin Pharmacol Appl Skin Physiol, **14**(Suppl. 1): 98–102.

Weigmann HJ, Lindemann U, Antoniou C, Tsikrikas GN, Stratigos AI, Katsambas A, Sterry W & Lademann J (2003) UV/VIS absorbance allows rapid, accurate, and reproducible mass determination of corneocytes removed by tape stripping. Skin Pharmacol Appl Skin Physiol, **16**(4): 217–227.

Weigmann HJ, Ulrich J, Schanzer S, Jacobi U, Schaefer H, Sterry W & Lademann J (2005) Comparison of transepidermal water loss and spectroscopic absorbance to quantify changes of the stratum corneum after tape stripping. Skin Pharmacol Physiol, **18**(4): 180–185.

Wellner T & Korinth G (2004) Percutaneous absorption of pyrene using in vitro microdialysis. In: Brain KR & Walters KA eds. Perspectives in percutaneous penetration. Vol. 9a. Abstracts of presentations at the ninth international perspectives in percutaneous penetration conference held in La Grande Motte, April 2004. Cardiff, STS Publishing, p 99.

Wertz PW, Swartzendruber DC, Madison KC & Downing DT (1987) Composition and morphology of epidermal cyst lipids. J Invest Dermatol, **89**: 419–425.

Wester RC & Maibach HI (1985) Structure–activity correlations in percutaneous absorption. In: Bronaugh RL & Maibach HI eds. Percutaneous absorption: mechanisms–methodology–drug delivery. New York, Marcel Dekker, pp 107–123.

Wester RC & Maibach HI (1996) Percutaneous absorption: short-term exposure, lag time, multiple exposures, model variations, and absorption from clothing. In: Marzulli FN & Maibach HI eds. Dermatotoxicology, 5th ed. Washington, DC, Hemisphere Publishing Corporation, pp 35–48.

Wester RC & Maibach HI (1999a) Regional variation in percutaneous absorption. In: Bronaugh RL & Maibach HI eds. Percutaneous absorption: drugs–cosmetics–mechanisms–methodology, 3rd ed. New York, Marcel Dekker, pp 107–116 (Drugs and the Pharmaceutical Sciences Vol. 97).

Wester RC & Maibach HI (1999b) Importance of in vivo percutaneous absorption measurements. In: Bronaugh RL & Maibach HI eds. Percutaneous absorption: drugs–cosmetics–mechanisms–methodology, 3rd ed. New York, Marcel Dekker, pp 215–227 (Drugs and the Pharmaceutical Sciences Vol. 97).

Wester RC, Maibach HI, Bucks DA & Guy RH (1983) Malathion percutaneous absorption after repeated administration to man. Toxicol Appl Pharmacol, **68**(1): 116–119.

Wester RC, Maibach HI, Melendres J, Sedik L, Knaak J & Wang R (1992) In vivo and in vitro percutaneous absorption and skin evaporation of isofenphos in man. Fundam Appl Toxicol, **19**(4): 521–526.

Wester RC, Melendres J, Sedik L & Maibach HI (1994) Percutaneous absorption of azone following single and multiple doses to human volunteers. J Pharm Sci, **83**: 124–125.

Wiechers JW (1989) The barrier function of the skin in relation to percutaneous absorption of drugs. Pharm Weekbl Sci, **11**: 185–198.

Wilkinson SC & Williams FM (2002) Effects of experimental conditions on absorption of glycol ethers through human skin in vitro. Int Arch Occup Environ Health, **75**(8): 519–527.

Wilkinson SC, Mass WJM, Nielsen JB, Greaves LC, van de Sandt JJM & Williams FM (2004) Influence of skin thickness on percutaneous penetration in vitro. In: Brain KR & Walters KA eds. Perspectives in percutaneous penetration. Vol. 9a. Abstracts of presentations at the ninth international perspectives in percutaneous penetration conference held in La Grande Motte, April 2004. Cardiff, STS Publishing, p 83.

Wilkinson SC, Maas WJ, Nielsen JB, Greaves LC, van de Sandt JJ & Williams FM (2006) Interactions of skin thickness and physicochemical properties of test compounds in percutaneous penetration studies. Int Arch Occup Environ Health, **79**(5): 405–413.

Williams FM (2004a) EDETOX. Evaluations and predictions of dermal absorption of toxic chemicals. Int Arch Occup Environ Health, **77**: 150–151.

Williams FM (2004b) Percutaneous penetration of occupationally relevant chemicals. In: Brain KR & Walters KA eds. Perspectives in percutaneous penetration. Vol. 9a. Abstracts of presentations at the ninth international perspectives in percutaneous penetration conference held in La Grande Motte, April 2004. Cardiff, STS Publishing, p 10.

Williams ML & Elias PM (2000) Ichthyosis: Where we have been; Disorders of cornification: Where we are going. Curr Probl Dermatol, **12**: 171–176.

Wilschut A, ten Berge WF, Robinson PJ & McKone TE (1995) Estimating skin permeation. The validation of five mathematical skin permeation models. Chemosphere, **30**(7): 1275–1296.

Wolfram LJ & Maibach HI (1985) Percutaneous penetration of hair dyes. Arch Dermatol Res, **277**: 235–241.

Woollen BH, Marsh JR, Laird WJ & Lesser JE (1992) The metabolism of cypermethrin in man: Differences in urinary metabolite profiles following oral and dermal absorption. Xenobiotica, **22**: 983–991.

World Medical Association (2004) Declaration of Helsinki: Ethical principles for medical research involving human subjects. Ferney-Voltaire, World Medical Association, pp 1–5 (http://www.wma.net).

Wurster DE & Kramer SF (1961) Investigation of some factors influencing percutaneous absorption. J Pharm Sci, **50**: 288–293.

Yang JJ, Roy TA & Mackerer CR (1986a) Percutaneous absorption of anthracene in the rat: comparison of in vivo and in vitro results. Toxicol Ind Health, **2**: 79–84.

Yang JJ, Roy TA & Mackerer CR (1986b) Percutaneous absorption of benzo[*a*]pyrene in the rat: comparison of in vivo and in vitro results. Toxicol Ind Health, **2**: 409–416.

Yano T, Nakagawa A, Tsuji M & Noda K (1986) Skin permeability of various non-steroidal anti-inflammatory drugs in man. Life Sci, **39**(12): 1043–1050.

Yourick JJ & Bronaugh RL (2000) Percutaneous penetration and metabolism of 2-nitro-*p*-phenylenediamine in human and fuzzy rat skin. Toxicol Appl Pharmacol, **166**(1): 13–23.

Yourick JJ, Koenig ML, Yourick DL & Bronaugh RL (2004) Fate of chemicals in skin after dermal application: does the in vitro skin reservoir affect the estimate of systemic absorption? Toxicol Appl Pharmacol, **195**(3): 309–320.

Yu Z, Schwartz JB, Sugita ET & Foehl HC (1996) Five modified numerical deconvolution methods for biopharmaceutics and pharmacokinetics studies. Biopharm Drug Dispos, **17**: 521–540.

Zendzian RP (2000) Dermal absorption of pesticides in the rat. Am Ind Hyg Assoc J, **61**: 473–483.

Zendzian RP (2003) Pesticide residue on/in the washed skin and its potential contribution to dermal toxicity. J Appl Toxicol, **23**(2): 121–136.

Zesch A & Schaefer H (1975) [Penetration of radioactive hydrocortisone in human skin from various ointment bases. II. In vivo experiments.] Arch Dermatol Forsch, **252**(4): 245–256 (in German).

Zhai H & Maibach HI (2001) Effects of skin occlusion on percutaneous absorption: an overview. Skin Pharmacol Appl Skin Physiol, **14**(1): 1–10.

Zhai H & Maibach HI (2002) Occlusion vs. skin barrier function. Skin Res Technol, **8**(1): 1–6.

APPENDIX 1: GUIDELINES AND PROTOCOLS

A1.1 Historical perspectives

Although methodology for and assessment of percutaneous absorption have been advancing for several decades, it is only comparatively recently that interest in this area has expanded from the drugs and cosmetics branches to the field of chemical risk assessment. In the last decade, a number of documents have been prepared, reviewed internationally, and published for various associations or regulatory bodies. The following is intended only as a short guide to the available publications, which have, in part, been stepping stones in the preparation of the OECD test guidelines (OECD, 2004a,b,c). Details are to be found in the original documents.

A1.2 ECETOC (European Centre for Ecotoxicology & Toxicology of Chemicals)

ECETOC (1993) was prepared and reviewed by experts in the field of percutaneous absorption on behalf of ECETOC. With emphasis on industrial chemicals rather than on drugs or cosmetics, this publication describes methods for studying percutaneous absorption, discusses the relevance of results when forming interspecies comparisons, and reviews the assessment of dermal exposure.

A1.3 ECVAM (European Centre for the Validation of Alternative Methods)

Howes et al. (1996) is the Report and Recommendations of the ECVAM Workshop, which was held in 1994. The participants comprised scientists from both academia and industry. The aim of the workshop was to review the status of in vivo and in vitro methods for studying dermal absorption at that time, with particular emphasis on recommending and optimizing in vitro methods to reduce the number of animals needed for testing.

The group noted that the regulatory requirements for submission of relevant data on dermal penetration varied worldwide, from the very demanding and precise in vivo (rat) protocols of the USEPA for dermal absorption of pesticides (e.g. USEPA, 1998) to absence of guidelines. In Europe, the requirement for percutaneous absorption data was usually fulfilled as part of the ADME studies (pharmacokinetics/toxicokinetics) undertaken for new chemicals, drugs, and pesticides, as well as experimental data on the delivery of drugs. There was/is increasing pressure on industry to reduce the number of animals used in safety testing.

The ECVAM Report discusses mechanisms and modelling of skin penetration, in vitro and in vivo methods for measuring percutaneous absorption, and skin metabolism.

A1.4 COLIPA (European Cosmetic Toiletry and Perfumery Association)

Owing to a potential ban on the use of animals in the testing of cosmetic products and their ingredients (6th amendment to the European Cosmetics Directive 93/35/EEC), a Task Force of COLIPA met in 1995 to develop test guidelines for in vitro assessment of dermal absorption and percutaneous penetration of cosmetic ingredients (Diembeck et al., 1999). This publication was the basis for further activities by the cosmetics industry (see also Steiling et al., 2001).

A1.5 SCCNFP (Scientific Committee on Cosmetic Products and Non-Food Products Intended for Consumers)

SCCNFP (2003a) contains notes of guidance for testing of cosmetic ingredients for their safety evaluation. Only one subchapter (3-4.4) is related specifically to dermal/percutaneous absorption.

The document points out the wide variety of terms used in definitions. For cosmetics, the SCCNFP makes a clear distinction between dermal absorption and dermal adsorption, the latter being defined as the amount of topically applied test substance present in or sticking to the stratum corneum. It is considered not to be systemically available and is excluded from the risk assessment for cosmetic products (see Diembeck et al., 1999; also Steiling et al., 2001).

Dermal/percutaneous absorption is defined as the amount of dermally applied substance remaining in the residual skin (excluding the stratum corneum) plus the amount of dermally applied substance that has transpassed the skin and is detected in the receptor fluid. The sum is considered to be systemically available (= dermal bioavailability) (see Diembeck et al., 1999).

Test formulations and concentrations tested should be an adequate representation of the final cosmetic products. In cases where dermal absorption studies are not available, a default value for dermal absorption of 100% is applied in the calculation of the margin of safety.

Details of SCCNFP basic criteria for in vitro testing of cosmetic ingredients are given in SCCNFP/0750/03 (SCCNFP, 2003b). The SCCNFP has also published guidance in particular on in vitro dermal absorption of cosmetic ingredients and its assessment (SCCNFP, 2003b).

A1.6 USEPA (United States Environmental Protection Agency)

A1.6.1 USEPA (1998)

USEPA (1998) is intended to meet testing requirements of the United States Federal Insecticide, Fungicide, and Rodenticide Act and the TSCA. The guideline has been designed and validated using the laboratory rat, and this is the required species for testing. Other animal species were considered but were rejected. It is recommended that the same strain of rat used for metabolism and toxicology studies be used for dermal absorption testing. For risk assessment, the absorption rates determined in the rat can be used as a "modest overestimate" of human dermal absorption or to perform a kinetic evaluation.

A1.6.2 USEPA (2004a)

In their Final Test Rule (USEPA, 2004a; update of USEPA, 1999) under section 4(a) of the TSCA, manufacturers, importers, and processors of 34 (formerly 47) chemical substances of interest to the Occupational Safety and Health Administration (OSHA) will be required to conduct in vitro dermal absorption rate testing. These dermal absorption rate data are to be used to support OSHA's development of "skin designations" for the chemical substances. For measuring the permeability constant (K_p), the test standard specifies the use of static or flow-through diffusion cells and non-viable human cadaver skin. It also requires the use of radiolabelled test substances unless the analytical methods used have an equivalent sensitivity. For compounds that may damage the skin with prolonged contact, a short-term absorption rate measurement is more appropriate. The six parameters (choice of membrane, preparation of membrane, diffusion cell design, temperature, testing hydrophobic chemicals, and vehicle) are similar for the determination of either of the two percutaneous absorption rate values. In contrast, the remaining two parameters (dose and study duration) are different for the two percutaneous absorption rate values.

A1.6.3 USEPA (1992)

Dermal Exposure Assessment Principles and Applications is an interim document and details procedures for estimating permeability coefficients of toxic chemicals and for evaluating the dermal absorbed dose. This is updated in USEPA (2004b).

A1.6.4 USEPA (2004b)

This document is the *Supplemental Guidance (Part E) to the Risk Assessment Guidance for Superfund, Volume 1: Human Health Evaluation Manual.* USEPA (2004b) incorporates and updates the USEPA (1992) document and contains methods for conducting dermal risk assessments for the water and soil pathways at Superfund sites. The USEPA has a web site where update information can be found (http://www.epa.gov/oswer/riskassessment).

The permeability factor K_p has been identified as one of the major parameters contributing to uncertainty in the assessment of dermal exposures. Since, according to this document, the variability between predicted and measured K_p values is no greater than the variability in interlaboratory replicated measurements, the USEPA (2004b) document recommends the use of a mathematical model to predict K_p values (given in Appendices A and B of that document) based on equations estimated via an empirical correlation as a function of K_{ow} and molecular weight (Potts & Guy, 1992), obtained from an experimental database (the Flynn [1990] data set) using absorption data of about 90 chemicals from water through human skin in vitro.

Based on the Flynn (1990) data set, Equation 3.8 (of the USEPA 2004b document) was derived and can be used to predict the K_p of chemicals with K_{ow} and molecular weight (MW) within the "Effective Prediction Domain" determined via a statistical analysis:

$$\text{Log } K_p = -2.80 + 0.66 \log K_{ow} - 0.0056 \text{ MW} \qquad (r^2 = 0.66)$$

However, there are some chemicals that fall outside the "Effective Prediction Domain" for determining K_p, in particular those with a high molecular weight and high K_{ow} values (lipophilic compounds accumulating in the stratum corneum). It is suggested in this document that a fraction absorbed term be applied to account for the loss of chemical due to desquamation of the outer skin layer and a corresponding reduction in the absorbed dermal dose. For halogenated chemicals, the predicted K_p could be underestimated due to the lower ratio of molar volume related to molecular weight compared with those included in the Flynn (1990) data set.

The USEPA (2004b) document gives a table (Exhibit B-2) of predicted K_p values for 209 organic chemical contaminants in water.

The USEPA (2004b) guidance document presents recommended default exposure values for all variables for the dermal–water and dermal–soil pathways.

For guidance on permeability coefficients for inorganic compounds, USEPA presents a table compiled from specific chemical experimental data as modified from USEPA (1992) and Hostynek et al. (1998).

A1.7 EC (European Commission)

A1.7.1 EC (2003)

In Appendix IVB of the EC Technical Guidance Document on Risk Assessment (EC, 2003), the contribution that dermal exposure may make to systemic body uptake and its estimation are discussed.

Although guidelines give a general description of the experimental design, it is important for risk assessment that the anticipated exposure conditions be taken into account (Benford et al., 1999).

The duration and frequency of exposure as well as the level of exposure may vary tremendously — exposure may be incidental or continuous. Studies addressing more than one relevant exposure per unit area are recommended, as well as the use of various exposure times and vehicles. For risk assessment, the percentage of absorption is the most useful parameter. Ideally, 1) the exposure duration of the study should be as long as or longer than the anticipated exposure duration, and 2) the concentrations tested should include the lowest concentration anticipated.

The Technical Guidance Document presents the problems encountered when making risk assessments 1) when studies are not available (default values) and 2) from in vitro and in vivo data. Some of this discussion is given in chapter 11 on risk assessment in the present report.

A1.7.2 EC (2004)

This guidance document on dermal absorption has been prepared for the EC Directorate E1 – Plant Health (EC, 2004). Therefore, the emphasis is on guidance for notifiers and EU Member States on the setting of dermal absorption values to be used in risk assessment for users of plant protection products reviewed for inclusion in Annex I of Directive 91/414/EEC. Inclusion of active substances in this annex is possible only if the products containing them can be used with acceptable risk to humans (i.e. operators, workers, bystanders). The dermal route is the main exposure route for most pesticides for operators applying them as well as for workers and bystanders.

The EC (2004) document contains an overview of dermal absorption and the methodologies used in measuring dermal absorption. It discusses the decision-making processes for setting absorption percentages and includes a proposal for a tiered approach to risk assessment for operator exposure, using default dermal absorption percentage or dermal absorption percentage determined experimentally (see also chapter 11 in the present report).

In the absence of experimental data, the occupational exposure is based on models — for example, the European Predictive Operator Exposure Model (EURO POEM; http://www.pesticides.gov.uk) — each calculating external dermal and inhalation exposure. For risk assessment, these external exposure data are compared with toxicity data (acceptable operator exposure level or AOEL, defined as an internal value and expressed in mg/kg body weight per day; EC, 2001). In order to compare the external exposure with the internal AOEL, external exposure data have to be converted into internal levels. The studies should be performed in accordance with OECD Test Guidelines 427 (OECD, 2004b) and 428 (OECD, 2004c) and the associated Guidance Document No. 28 (OECD, 2004a).

A1.8 OECD (Organisation for Economic Co-operation and Development)

A1.8.1 OECD (2004a)

This guidance document was written to guide scientists unfamiliar with the procedures of skin absorption studies and to support technical aspects of the OECD skin absorption test guidelines (OECD, 2004b,c).

A1.8.2 OECD (2004b)

This guideline describes details of the in vivo studies commonly performed on rats but also on hairless species as well as other species having skin absorption rates more similar to those of humans.

A1.8.3 OECD (2004c)

This guideline describes in vitro methods used for studying dermal absorption. Skin from human or laboratory animal sources can be used. It is recognized that the use of human skin is subject to national and international ethical considerations and conditions. Both static and flow-through diffusion cells are acceptable. Normally, donor chambers are left unoccluded during exposure to a finite dose of a test preparation. However, for some studies, infinite applications are necessary when donor chambers may be occluded (see also chapter 6).

APPENDIX 2: PAST AND PRESENT INITIATIVES ON EXCHANGE OF INFORMATION AND HARMONIZATION OF METHODOLOGY ON DERMAL ABSORPTION

In the last few years, there have been several initiatives to accelerate progress in international harmonization of methodology and protocols of dermal absorption, culminating in the publication of the OECD test guidelines in 2004 (OECD, 2004a,b,c; see Appendix 1).

There have been initiatives from the regulatory side in the United States (USEPA, 1999, 2004a,b) and in Europe. In Europe, there have been two large projects: the Dermal Exposure Network (1997–1999) and, leading on from it, the EDETOX project. From the industrial side, CEFIC has supported two projects associated with QSARs linking 1) physicochemical properties to permeation data and 2) measured with calculated values, so that in the future it may be possible to predict the data for a large number of chemicals rather than undertake expensive testing of chemicals. Here, an overview is given of these projects, the results of which are also cited in other parts of the document.

In addition, it should be emphasized that this interest and progress in dermal absorption harmonization have been a result of the momentum from the biannual meetings of the Prediction of Percutaneous Penetration (PPP) Conferences (later the Perspectives in Percutaneous Penetration Conferences; section A2.5) and Gordon Research Conferences (section A2.6) and, more recently, the International Conference on Occupational and Environmental Exposures of Skin to Chemicals (section A2.7).

A2.1 OECD Test Guidelines

The most important recent international initiative was the effort to harmonize the protocols for in vitro and in vivo testing (see also chapters 6 and 7 and Appendix 1). The need for a guidance document became apparent in 1997 when national experts from a number of member countries could not agree on the possibilities and limitations of the in vitro test. The draft outlines were presented in 2000, and the final guidelines were published in 2004 (OECD, 2004a,b,c). The guidance document (OECD, 2004a) provides additional technical background to both the in vivo and in vitro methods for skin absorption, as described in Test Guidelines 427 (OECD, 2004b) and 428 (OECD, 2004c), respectively.

A2.2 Dermal Exposure Network (1997–1999)

At an international meeting of experts from European countries and the United States in June 1994, it was decided to form a European network on dermal exposure to encourage development of projects in the area and pool research capabilities, to harmonize techniques, expertise, and knowledge, and to guide the EC in developing a comprehensive and harmonized risk assessment strategy in the workplace. Under the Environment and Health Programme of the EC, the Dermal Exposure Network was established, with members comprising skin experts from many countries in Europe. Meetings of the Dermal Exposure Network of the EC started in 1997, and five subgroups were organized: Risk Assessment, Biological Monitoring, Percutaneous Penetration, Skin and Surface Contamination, and Contribution of Different Sources (Sartorelli et al., 2000).

The work of the Percutaneous Penetration Subgroup of the Dermal Exposure Network focused on the standardization and validation of in vitro experiments necessary to obtain internationally accepted penetration rates for regulatory purposes. The key items discussed were:

- the use of percutaneous penetration data in risk assessment;
- in in vitro studies, the factors influencing
  - the choice of cell characteristics,
  - the choice of donor phase,
  - receptor fluids;
- the presentation of in vitro percutaneous penetration results;
- existing guidelines on in vitro percutaneous penetration studies;
- prediction of plasma levels from penetration data;
- the influence of cutaneous metabolism on skin absorption;

- criteria for the selection of reference compounds for in vitro percutaneous penetration;
- the use of microdialysis for the determination of percutaneous penetration of hazardous substances in vivo; and
- correlation between in vitro and in vivo experiments.

The members of the Percutaneous Penetration Subgroup analysed the guidelines on in vitro percutaneous penetration studies presented by various organizations and suggested a standardization of in vitro models for percutaneous penetration taking into account their individual experiences, literature data, and guidelines already in existence. The subgroup also presented a number of short papers of up-to-date information on the key issues to focus the existing knowledge and knowledge gaps in the field of percutaneous penetration. The publication (Sartorelli et al., 2000) is an outcome of work of this subgroup during the Dermal Exposure Network Project (1997–1999).

From this network, two research projects developed that were funded by the EU. These were RISKOFDERM dermal exposure monitoring and EDETOX. Within RISKOFDERM: Risk Assessment of Occupational Dermal Exposure to Chemicals, 15 European institutes/organizations from 10 European member states worked together with the following major aims (van Hemmen et al., 2003; van Hemmen, 2004):

- to develop a validated/benchmarked predictive model for estimating dermal exposure for use in generic risk assessment for single chemicals; and
- to develop a practical dermal exposure risk assessment and management toolkit for use by small and medium-sized enterprises, and others, in actual workplace situations.

A predictive model for dermal exposure assessment was produced based on the conceptual model for dermal exposure of Schneider et al. (1999) (Marquart et al., 2003). In a further part of the project, a toolkit for hazard, exposure, and risk assessment of dermal exposure based on label information and material safety data sheets was developed (Oppl et al., 2003). During this project, a series of quantitative dermal exposure measurements were carried out (references published in *Annals of Occupational Hygiene*,

Volume 48, Number 3, 2004). The next step would be to implement the results in European regulations on notification of chemicals in current frameworks and for workplace risk assessments of chemical compounds.

A2.3 EDETOX (Evaluations and Predictions of Dermal Absorption of Toxic Chemicals)

EDETOX was a 3-year multipartner EU project (2001–2003/4) funded under the Framework V Programme to generate new data on dermal absorption of chemicals (EDETOX, undated). The consortium comprised 12 participants from seven EU member states. The project aimed to define robustness and standardize in vitro systems for predicting percutaneous penetration and to compare these with relevant in vivo studies, mainly in humans. It also aimed to use the standardized in vitro methods to generate occupationally relevant dermal absorption data acceptable for risk assessment and data to evaluate QSARs and predictive models of skin penetration of health-related chemicals. A database of evaluated literature and data generated during the project has been established and used in the QSAR and predictive models (Williams, 2004a,b). The results of the EDETOX project were presented in a research day at the Perspectives in Percutaneous Penetration conference in 2004 (see section A2.5). The full report of the EDETOX project is completed, and a summary is available at http://www.ncl.ac.uk/edetox (EDETOX, 2004). An updated list of publications is available on the web site.

A2.3.1 Work package 1: Robustness of in vitro methodology

2.3.1.1 Intra- and interlaboratory variation in in vitro dermal absorption methodology

A major part of the EDETOX project was a study into the intra- and interlaboratory variation in dermal absorption data generated by in vitro methods The dermal absorptions of benzoic acid, caffeine, and testosterone were determined following a detailed protocol using human skin (nine laboratories) and rat skin (one laboratory) (EDETOX, 2004; van de Sandt, 2004). There was some variability between the results due, to a large extent, to interindividual variability in absorption between samples of human skin. The results are discussed in chapter 8. The observations from this study stimulated further investigations of particular aspects of optimization of experimental conditions.

A2.3.1.2 Effects of experimental conditions on dermal absorption

The influence of skin thickness on percutaneous penetration of caffeine, testosterone, butoxyethanol, and propoxur through human skin in vitro was investigated (Wilkinson et al., 2004). Skin thickness influenced the absorption rate of lipophilic molecules to a greater extent than that of less lipophilic molecules. Physicochemical properties must be taken into account when considering skin preparation.

In vivo (rodent) and in vitro (human and rodent) absorption data generated for five pesticides of varying lipophilicity in a range of formulations were considered to assess the contribution of the stratum corneum reservoir to absorbed chemical for risk estimations. Inclusion of the material remaining in the stratum corneum appeared to overpredict the level of absorption in vivo when using the recommended in vivo/in vitro calculation (O'Connor & Cage, 2004; O'Connor et al., 2004) (see chapters 6 and 12).

A2.3.2 Work package 2: In vivo studies in volunteers

A2.3.2.1 Human in vivo studies of dermal absorption: their relation to in vitro prediction

Human in vivo studies have served as the gold standard to evaluate in vitro results. For a range of chemicals of different physicochemical properties (2-butoxyethanol [aqueous solutions of different composition], trichloroethene, *m*-xylene vapour, and caffeine), the percutaneous absorption was determined in parallel in human volunteers and in vitro with human skin using the same dose, vehicle, and application time (EDETOX, 2004; Kezic, 2004). The percutaneous absorption of 2-butoxyethanol from aqueous solution was much higher than that of neat 2-butoxyethanol (Jakasa et al., 2004b), and this was predicted from the parallel in vitro studies. In volunteer studies, dermal absorption was determined using two different methods: microdialysis and biomonitoring. The comparison of 2-butoxyethanol data between the laboratories performing the in vivo experiments in volunteers showed good agreement; the apparent steady-state flux differed by a factor of 2. The correlation between in vivo and in vitro data was good (see chapters 6, 7, and 8). Parallel in vivo/in vitro studies with butoxyethanol, pyrene, benzo[*a*]pyrene, and di(2-ethylhexyl)phthalate at a range of concentrations were conducted in the rat (Kezic, 2004).

Parallel studies in which dermal microdialysis and urinary metabolite excretion were determined following application of 50% butoxyethanol in water were also conducted. Microdialysis studies of dermal absorption of pyrene in volunteers were compared with in vitro studies. The microdialysis technique has been modified for in vitro tests — e.g. studying the absorption of three low molecular weight (radiolabelled) test compounds (toluene, 50% aqueous butoxyethanol, and propoxur) using glass diffusion cells (Maas et al., 2004). In a further experiment, an infinite dose of non-radiolabelled pyrene in ethanol was investigated using in vitro microdialysis (Wellner & Korinth, 2004).

A2.3.3 Work package 3: In vitro measurement of dermal absorption

In the EDETOX project, finite dose data were generated for 60 chemicals at occupationally relevant exposures using the previously standardized guidelines for in vitro studies. Chemicals chosen were from classes for which dermal absorption may pose a risk and risk assessment will be required. New data included effect of sweat on absorption of metal, effect of water on butoxyethanol dermal absorption, effect of vehicle on caffeine and pesticide absorption, dermal absorption data for an extended series of glycol ethers, natural oils, and pesticides, and absorption and metabolism of aromatic amines (EDETOX, 2004).

2.3.3.1 *In vitro dermal absorption of metals*

Studies into the in vitro percutaneous absorption of metal powders (nickel, cobalt, and chromium) (Venier et al., 2004) showed that metallic ions can easily permeate the skin. Using the Franz cell, it was possible to measure a flux of ions through the skin for cobalt and nickel but not for chromium (Larese Filon et al., 2004). A similar study was described by Sartorelli et al. (2004). Synthetic sweat promoted the absorption of metals through the skin.

A2.3.3.2 *Dermal absorption of pesticides*

In an in vitro percutaneous penetration study of five pesticides covering a range of solubilities and molecular weights, it was shown that molecular weight as well as solubility affect dermal penetration. After short-term occupational exposures, an exposure assessment based on penetrated pesticide at the end of the work shift may underestimate the exposure. This suggests that data used by the regulatory agencies should include maximum flux (or K_p), lag time, as well as an estimation of the potential importance of the skin reservoir (Nielsen et al., 2004a,b). Further studies on pesticides are in the process of publication.

A2.3.3.3 *Dermal absorption of aromatic amines*

Absorption and local metabolism and adduct formation of aromatic amines such as trimethylamine (Kenyon et al., 2004a) and 4,4'-methylenedianiline (Kenyon et al., 2004b) were studied.

A2.3.4 *Work package 4: Modelling and prediction of absorption*

A2.3.4.1 *EDETOX database*

A database has been compiled giving details of in vitro and in vivo studies on percutaneous penetration of chemicals. This database is freely available on the EDETOX web site (http://www.ncl.ac.uk/edetox). The purpose of the database was to compile in vivo and in vitro percutaneous absorption and distribution data from all available sources together with the physicochemical data for each chemical for use in occupational risk assessment. The database currently contains 4800 studies for 320 chemicals. Data have been assessed against specific inclusion criteria. Less than half of the studies satisfied the criteria for required details (Soyei & Williams, 2004).

A2.3.4.2 *Modelling of dermal absorption*

Because of the complex nature of the skin membrane, the modelling of dermal absorption was confined to 1) QSARs that relate the dermal absorption of a molecule to some of its physicochemical properties and 2) the modelling of the macroscopic behaviour of the absorption process using diffusion equations or compartmental models.

1) QSARs for dermal absorption

Existing QSARs for percutaneous penetration were evaluated (Fitzpatrick et al., 2004; Golden et al., 2004). Infinite dose (saturated aqueous) data were generated for 21 chemicals for comparison with the data set gathered by Flynn (1990) or by Cronin et al. (1999) as the basis of predictive QSAR models used today. It was identified that there was a need for further investigations of the effect of vehicle, formulation, multiple doses, and mixtures on absorption.

2) Further modelling of dermal absorption data

Another approach has been to model the absorption process using diffusion equations or compartmental models that represent the vehicle, the sink, and the various layers of the skin (Corish, 2004). A comparative analysis of non-steady-state data using two diffusion models has been presented (Corish et al., 2004; Krüse & Kezic, 2004).

A mechanistically based mathematical model was developed during the project, which was used to interpret infinite and finite absorption data for triclosan, malathion, testosterone, parathion, and caffeine (Corish et al., 2004; J. Krüse, unpublished data, 2006). This model enables the time courses of various variables to be simulated, and modelling of a variety of exposure regimes, such as single and multiple dosing from different application forms, can be handled. The development of these models and their testing through application to data measured in the EDETOX project have resulted in considerable progress towards the development of a more reliable predictive tool for the estimation of the extent of dermal penetration of a chemical based on its physicochemical properties.

A2.3.5 Work package 5: Dissemination of results and discussion of skin notation

A2.3.5.1 Recommendations from EDETOX (htp://www.ncl.ac.uk/edetox)

The EDETOX project showed that outcomes from both predictive modelling and the design of in vitro protocols influence generation of data suitable for improving existing QSAR models and building novel models for dermal absorption. EDETOX recommended a refinement of the in vitro protocol and generation of further data to improve QSARs. This has also been highlighted by CEFIC (see section A2.4).

EDETOX found that there was a need for further investigations of the effect of vehicle, formulation, multiple doses, and mixtures on absorption and suggested that data should be generated for QSARs that take into account the effect of vehicles.

Further work was recommended in the area of an EU-wide skin notation system that might be semiquantitative.

Further research is required to identify and define factors contributing to interindividual variability in dermal absorption in order to be able to predict how permeable an individual's skin might be.

The importance of local metabolism and generation of toxic metabolites producing local skin damage such as irritation and sensitization following penetration was emphasized and should be further investigated.

EDETOX recommended that future research should concentrate on development of finite dose models to mathematically define the profile of dermal penetration through skin both in vitro and in vivo at exposure relevant to low-level, short-term doses. These should be extended to investigate the effects of multiple exposures, exposure to mixtures, and vehicle and formulation effects on the dermal absorption profile of chemicals. It is important to compare finite and infinite doses and effects of vehicles on the absorption profile in detail to provide a database of information with which to validate this model.

EDETOX recommended that the use of the direct modelling approach should be pursued to assess its use for risk assessment in areas such as the new EU REACH regulations on use of chemicals.

The EDETOX project concentrated on the use of human skin in in vitro systems, as results with this can be directly extrapolated to risk assessment for humans. However, with reduced availability of human skin for investigation due to ethical issues, further investigations of alternatives such as pig or rodent skin should be initiated.

A2.3.5.2 *Skin notation*

Preliminary discussions were held on skin notation concerning a) the strengths and weaknesses of the present approach to the use of skin notations in different EU and non-EU countries and b) possible ways of refining the skin notation in order to make it usable for prevention in occupational settings (Nielsen & Grandjean, 2004; Nielsen et al., 2004c).

A2.4 European Chemical Industry Council (CEFIC) initiatives

A2.4.1 Determination of the optimal physicochemical parameters to use in a QSAR approach to predict skin permeation rate

Approaches funded by CEFIC and previously published (Patel & Cronin, 2001; Moss et al., 2002; Patel et al., 2002) were considered at the workshop and have been discussed in chapter 10 of this document.

A2.4.2 CEFIC workshop on methods to determine dermal permeation for human risk assessment (Utrecht, 13–15 June 2004) (taken from Jones et al., 2004)

A2.4.2.1 *Introduction*

The proposed new European chemicals strategy involving the Registration, Evaluation, Authorisation and Restriction of Chemicals (REACH) is likely to involve 10 000 industrial chemicals and many more mixtures. Data on the potential for dermal uptake are available for only a small number of these chemicals, and these were often obtained not using a standardized protocol. Obtaining human in vivo or in vitro data on all REACH chemicals is not feasible. The European Chemical Industry (through CEFIC, the European Chemical Industry Council) recognized the need to establish a systematic tiered approach to predict dermal permeation of chemicals for risk assessment.

With this in mind, a meeting sponsored by the CEFIC Long-range Research Initiative (LRI) was convened to reach a consensus on methods to determine dermal absorption in vitro, and it was intended that data produced from a limited number of these studies would be used to develop a QSAR linking physicochemical properties to permeation data so that, ideally, it would be possible to predict the data for a large number of chemicals rather than undertake expensive testing.

Approximately 20 experts in skin permeation, risk assessment, and QSAR were invited from academia, contract testing laboratories, industry, regulatory agencies, and the EC. At the meeting, presentations and discussions spanned the assessment of dermal exposure, permeation measurements in the laboratory, and the application of permeation data to risk assessment and brought together the views from two preceding conferences: the April 2004 PPP Conference and a 2004 QSAR meeting (11th International Workshop on Quantitative Structure–Activity Relationships in the Human Health and Environmental Sciences, 9–13 May, Liverpool, England; http://www.cefic-lri.org).

Before the meeting, there had been concerns that the QSAR predictions that had previously been made might be unreliable, as they had been based on in vitro tests conducted using a variety of methods over more than a decade. However, discussions at the meeting led to the conclusion that the existing databases for K_p, despite some inherent variability due to methodological differences, were acceptable for derivation of the existing QSARs. Further, it was not expected that further data would produce any significant revision of the QSARs. However, it was recognized that the existing database was primarily from chemicals from specialized sectors or selected on the basis of physicochemical properties, and the meeting recommended that generation of in vitro data and K_p for a range of relevant industrial chemicals would be valuable in reassuring all stakeholders of the validity and relevance of QSARs within the broad application area of REACH. Chemicals should be selected as being of greatest relevance to high volume production chemical manufacture and should provide a good coverage of the range of physicochemical properties needed to produce data that will support the development of QSAR models.

Further to this was the discussion of the relevance of infinite dose studies to realistic risk assessment scenarios, which usually correspond to finite dose conditions. Data used for QSARs have up to now been those from infinite in vitro assays, which are most suitable for establishing a stable maximum flux and calculating a permeability coefficient K_p, and which can be related by QSARs to physicochemical properties.

Therefore, a link must be established between finite and infinite dose experiments, thus linking the QSAR-derived information with the inputs required for risk assessment. This link relies on mathematical modelling, which requires that a sound theoretical basis is used in the interpretation of data from each experiment and should improve the reliability of parameters calculated from experimental data. The model also enables extrapolation to predict absorption under different dosing conditions.

In a further contribution, data for a range of pesticides were presented, which showed how predictions of absorption (based on QSAR-predicted K_p) compare with systemic absorption in vivo measured in rats (Zendzian, 2000; Reddy & Bunge, 2002). Such data could be used to predict a safety factor such that the safety factor multiplied by the predicted systemic absorption would encompass the majority of the set of measured values for the in vivo systemic absorption.

A2.4.2.2 Proposed finite and infinite dose protocols (Appendices 2 and 3 of the CEFIC protocol)

These protocols have been suggested as the most effective and timely way of obtaining data robust enough to construct a QSAR model that could be acceptable to all interest groups.

A2.4.2.3 *Chemicals to be selected for testing*

The following recommendations were made to CEFIC by the meeting members for the selection of chemicals for developing the acceptance of QSARs as a valid and reliable method of predicting the permeability for industrial chemicals:

- The chemicals should span the physicochemical space of the parameters log K_{ow} from −3 to 7 and molecular weight from 30 to 1000 (an elliptical space on a two-dimensional plot of chemicals by these two parameters).
- The chemicals should be chosen from chemicals that are produced in high volume in industry.
- The chemicals should be chosen in conjunction with industry.
- If possible, the chemicals should be radiolabelled versions of the production chemicals (by selecting chemicals for which radioactive versions are available).
- If some non-radiolabelled chemicals are used (to obtain the range of physicochemical characteristics), then the chosen chemicals need to be suitable for sensitive chemical analysis.

A2.4.2.4 *Strategy recommendations*

The CEFIC Workshop recommended a two-stage strategy:

- **Stage 1** — Build on an already extensive data set for aqueous soluble chemicals and the QSARs that have been made for these chemicals.

  1) To promote the recognition of the likely reliability of QSAR predictions of dermal permeation for industrial chemicals. The CEFIC Workshop suggested a project measuring the permeation of a selection of about 50 chemicals using the proposed infinite dose protocol.
  2) To establish the validity of using the mathematical models to extrapolate from infinite dose to finite dose. The model should be used to extrapolate from infinite dose to predict

the results of a finite dose experiment before the results of the finite dose experiment are available.

It is important, especially for QSAR, that variability be minimized. Recent studies concerning robustness and variability (van de Sandt, 2004; Chilcott et al., 2005) have highlighted the problems that still exist in the field of in vitro dermal absorption measurements.

The CEFIC Workshop recommended that the first stage would use a wide range of chemicals with the standard aqueous solution protocol. The data from this project would be directly comparable with those of the existing data set already used for the development of QSARs and could be extrapolated using mathematical models for comparisons with finite dose data.

- **Stage 2** of the CEFIC Workshop recommendations involves more detailed testing of those chemicals in subset 1 together with more lipophilic chemicals that cannot be tested in the aqueous solution protocol. Further, there would be investigations into the effects of various donor fluids, receptor fluids, and mixtures.

The aim is to facilitate the development of models bridging the results from Stage 1 (standard aqueous solution test conditions) to Stage 2 (more complex and more realistic exposure conditions for an extended range of chemicals). A further objective would be a standardized protocol for chemicals in solution in other liquids.

A2.4.2.5 *Recommendations of CEFIC Workshop for use of their proposed new data in risk assessments*

1) Assume either 100% absorption or 10% default assumption for high molecular weight and log K_{ow} <-1 or >4; and then, if necessary,
2) Use saturated water concentration and K_p to calculate an estimate of maximum flux, allowing for any effects from the vehicle; then, if necessary,
3) Use the more complete mathematical model with diffusion coefficients and partition coefficients to obtain a best estimate

of the flux and dose for the likely occupational exposure concentration (i.e. finite dose).

Future developments in determining dermal permeation should be conducted in close liaison with developments in dermal exposure assessment (Kromhout et al., 2004; Semple, 2004).

A2.5 Perspectives in Percutaneous Penetration (PPP) Conferences

The purpose of the Perspectives in Percutaneous Penetration (formerly Prediction of Percutaneous Penetration) or PPP Conferences is to provide a forum for the presentation and discussion of all the latest research, development, and technology concerning the penetration of exogenous compounds through the skin. The meetings are of relevance and interest to those involved in dermatological research, the development of formulations, risk assessment, and regulatory affairs relating to the dermal effects of molecules within the agrochemical, cosmetic, and pharmaceutical fields within industrial, academic, and governmental domains. The PPP Conferences are biannual (http://www.pppconference.org).

The first Prediction of Percutaneous Penetration Conference took place in Manchester, United Kingdom, in 1989, the second conference in Southampton, United Kingdom, in 1991, and the third and fourth in La Grande Motte, France, in 1993 and 1995. Subsequently, the conference was renamed Perspectives in Percutaneous Penetration, and conferences have taken place in 1997, 1998, 2000, 2002, and 2004. Proceedings of the first five conferences were published in full (Scott et al., 1990, 1991b; Brain et al., 1993, 1996, 1998b), but the later conference publications (Vol. 6b [1998], Vol. 7b [2000], Vol. 8b [2002], Vol. 9a [2004]) were abstracts only. The 10th conference is to be held in April 2006 in La Grande Motte.

A2.6 Gordon Research Conferences

The Gordon Research Conferences provide an international forum for the presentation and discussion of frontier research in the biological, chemical, and physical sciences and their related technologies. The Gordon Research Conferences on the "Barrier Function of Mammalian Skin" were established in 1989 to provide an interdisciplinary scientific forum focusing on the development, structure, and function of the barrier of mammalian skin. The conferences take place every 2 years (e.g. 1999, 2001, 2003, 2005). The next conference is scheduled for August 2007 in Rhode Island, USA. The programme of lectures and speakers for the last 10 years can be found through the Gordon Research Conferences' home page (http://www.grc.uri.edu).

A2.7 International Conference on Occupational and Environmental Exposures of Skin to Chemicals

The first meeting (September 2002) in Washington, DC, USA, was organized by the National Institute for Occupational Safety and Health and was convened to bring together scientists with many areas of expertise (dermatologists, occupational hygienists, laboratory researchers, policy-makers, and occupational physicians) to focus on the science, knowledge gaps, and policy opportunities related to occupational and environmental exposures of the skin to chemicals (Chen & Sartorelli, 2005).

A second meeting was held in June 2005 in Stockholm, Sweden (http://www.cdc.gov/niosh/topics/skin/OEESC2). A plenary session and a workshop were held for each of six themes: 1) Irritants and Wet Work, 2) Quantitative Risk Assessment, 3) Exposure Reduction, 4) Process-Based, Qualitative Risk Assessment, 5) Systemic Toxics, and 6) Allergens.

RESUME

On désigne par l'expression générale de résorption ou d'absorption dermique, cutanée ou percutanée le transport de substances chimiques de la surface externe de la peau vers l'intérieur du revêtement cutané et la circulation générale. Le présent document de la série des *Critères d'hygiène de l'environnement* donne une vue d'ensemble de l'absorption percutanée et de son application à l'évaluation du risque que représentent les substances chimiques. Il expose et analyse en outre un certain nombre de points intéressants concernant l'absorption percutanée. Celle-ci peut se produire à l'occasion d'une exposition à des substances chimiques, à des cosmétiques ou à des produits pharmaceutiques lors de l'exercice d'une activité professionnelle, dans l'environnement ou encore lorsqu'un consommateur expose sa peau à des produits de ce genre.

Membrane vivante, la peau est un organe complexe. Elle assure des fonctions de protection, de régulation de la température centrale et des pertes en eau, de défense et de réparation. La peau est constituée d'une région externe, l'épiderme, et d'une région interne, le derme. L'épiderme comporte diverses couches cellulaires dont la plus extérieure, appelée *stratum corneum* ou couche cornée, représente la principale barrière à la pénétration des substances chimiques étrangères. Lorsqu'il est fonctionnel, l'épiderme est capable de métaboliser les substances chimiques qui traversent la couche cornée. Le derme, qui sert de substrat physiologique à l'épiderme avasculaire, est parcouru par les vaisseaux sanguins, les nerfs sensitifs et les vaisseaux lymphatiques cutanés. La peau comporte également un certain nombre d'annexes telles que les follicules pileux ou encore les glandes sudoripares et les glandes sébacées qui prennent naissance dans le derme sous-papillaire.

La mesure de la perméabilité cutanée donne des résultats extrêmement variables. Les différences peuvent être considérables d'une espèce à l'autre. On sait peu de choses au sujet des variations en fonction de l'âge, sinon que la structure du revêtement cutané évolue avec celui-ci; en revanche, il ne semble pas que la perméabilité cutanée varie avec le sexe ou l'appartenance ethnique. La résorption percutanée dépend également de la localisation anatomique, de l'état du tégument et de son degré d'hydratation.

Au nombre des facteurs qui jouent un rôle dans l'absorption percutanée figurent : 1) les propriétés physico-chimiques de la substance étudiée; 2) les propriétés physico-chimiques et autres du véhicule dans lequel cette substance est dissoute; 3) les interactions entre la substance étudiée et le revêtement cutané; 4) les propriétés de la peau et le métabolisme cutané; 5) certains facteurs liés au système d'épreuve dans lequel s'effectue la mesure – par exemple, dose et volume de la substance étudiée, occlusion ou non occlusion du territoire cutané étudié, système d'épreuve in vitro ou in vivo ou encore durée d'exposition.

Des équations et des modèles théoriques ont été établis pour rendre compte du transport d'une substance chimique qui diffuse à travers la peau. En règle générale, le flux en régime stationnaire (J_{ss}) et le coefficient de perméabilité (K_p) sont les principaux paramètres que l'on détermine dans les tests in vitro au cours desquels on s'arrange pour que la concentration de la substance pénétrante assure le maintien d'une valeur constante (infinie) de la dose. On admet désormais que la détermination du flux maximum, du temps nécessaire pour que le flux atteigne sa valeur maximale, du temps de réaction, des teneurs résiduelles retenues dans la couche cornée et du bilan massique dans des conditions d'application « réelles » sont de première importance pour l'estimation de l'exposition.

La mesure du métabolisme d'une substance chimique en contact avec la peau peut être importante pour l'évaluation de la sécurité comme de l'efficacité. Certaines substances peuvent être métabolisées de manière appréciable lors de la résorption intradermique, processus qui peut conduire à la formation de métabolites actifs ou inactifs. Il est donc important de mesurer cette métabolisation pour une bonne évaluation de la sécurité. On a montré que des produits chimiques toxiques comme le benzo[*a*]pyrène subissaient une activation cutanée, d'autres substances étant susceptibles d'être hydrolysées ou conjuguées dans le derme avec pour conséquence une moindre disponibilité dans l'organisme. En général, il est possible de conserver sa viabilité à un échantillon de peau placé dans une cellule de diffusion in vitro à condition d'utiliser un tégument frais et un tampon physiologique. Il est recommandé de vérifier la viabilité de l'échantillon en mesurant l'activité des enzymes de métabolisation appropriées.

Les paramètres qui caractérisent la perméabilité de la couche cornée restent, pour la plupart, inchangés lorsqu'un échantillon est prélevé sur le corps. Il s'ensuit qu'il existe une bonne corrélation entre les mesures effectuées in vitro et in vivo sur les mêmes substances chimiques (du moins dans le cas de substances hydrophiles). Les tests in vitro peuvent être valablement substituées aux tests in vivo et présentent un certain nombre d'avantages par rapport à l'expérimentation sur des animaux entiers ou sur des sujets humains volontaires. Les méthodes in vitro mesurent la diffusion des substances chimiques dans et à travers la peau jusqu'à un compartiment liquidien et on peut utiliser des échantillons non viables pour mesurer uniquement la diffusion ou des échantillons fraîchement prélevés et métaboliquement actifs pour déterminer simultanément la diffusion et la métabolisation intradermique. La ligne directrice expérimentale 428 de l'Organisation pour la coopération et le développement économiques (OCDE) préconise l'harmonisation des méthodes de mesure. Outre ceux qui sont indiqués plus haut, d'autres facteurs expérimentaux influent sur l'absorption percutanée in vitro, à savoir l'épaisseur de l'échantillon de peau, les variations de température à l'intérieur du système d'épreuve et la composition du liquide récepteur. On peut utiliser des cellules de diffusion statiques ou à écoulement continu. Il existe aussi d'autres techniques, qui nécessitent des dispositifs plus élaborés, telles que le prélèvement par ruban adhésif ou l'utilisation d'une peau artificielle ou reconstituée.

Les méthodes in vivo permettent de déterminer la résorption percutanée de la substance étudiée ainsi que son passage dans l'organisme. Ces études in vivo ont, par rapport aux tests in vitro, le principal avantage d'utiliser un système d'épreuve physiologiquement et métaboliquement intact. Les études de pénétration percutanée effectuées in vivo utilisent des animaux de laboratoire, des rongeurs en général, mais peuvent également être pratiquées sur des sujets humains volontaires. Cette expérimentation sur volontaires humains est largement pratiquée pour l'étude des produits pharmaceutiques et, dans une moindre mesure, d'autres produits chimiques. Sur le plan méthodologique, le nec plus ultra est l'expérimentation humaine. Toutefois, toute étude in vivo soulève des questions d'ordre éthique. Le principal inconvénient de l'expérimentation sur animaux de laboratoire tient au fait qu'ils ont une perméabilité cutanée et une absorption systémique différentes de celles de l'Homme.

Des études sur volontaires humains montrent que l'exposition professionnelle à des liquides (solvants, par exemple) peut entraîner une très forte absorption percutanée. L'absorption percutanée par exposition à des vapeurs peut contribuer de manière importante à l'absorption totale de certains produits volatils, comme les éthers de glycol.

Les résultats d'études in vitro sur l'absorption percutanée sont de plus en plus souvent communiqués aux autorités responsables en vue de l'homologation de produits chimiques industriels, de cosmétiques ou encore de produits phytiatriques ou phytopharmaceutiques. De nombreuses études comparant l'absorption percutanée in vitro et in vivo chez l'Homme et l'animal ont été publiées. Lorsqu'elles sont correctement effectuées en suivant les lignes directrices de l'OCDE pour ce genre d'expérimentation, les études in vitro permettent une bonne prévision de l'absorption in vivo.

On a accumulé depuis plusieurs décennies une somme importante de données relatives à la pénétration percutanée de nombreux produits chimiques, pesticides, cosmétiques et produits pharmaceutiques. Ces données résultent d'études sur volontaires humains, d'expérimentations in vivo sur modèles animaux, d'études in vitro utilisant des échantillons de peau prélevés par exemple sur des sujets humains, des rongeurs, des porcs ou des cobayes et, plus récemment, d'études in vitro sur peau synthétique.

Au cours des cinquante dernières années, on a tenté, à maintes reprises, de faire des prévisions au sujet de la vitesse et de l'ampleur de l'absorption percutanée de manière à réduire les études in vitro ou in vivo nécessaires. C'est là un besoin encore plus important au vu de la multiplication des problèmes d'éthique posés par l'expérimentation humaine et animale comme d'ailleurs des considérations d'ordre économique et chronologique imposées par la réglementation. Les relations quantitatives structure-perméabilité (RQSP) sont des relations de nature statistique entre le flux en régime stationnaire d'un composé donné et divers descripteurs physicochimiques ou propriétés structurales de la molécule. Les relations quantitatives structure-activité (RQSA) sont également prises en compte dans les considérations relatives à la sécurité et à l'efficacité, notamment en ce qui concerne l'irritation, la sensibilisation cutanée, le métabolisme, les effets chimiques et la clairance. Les RQSA interviennent donc à plusieurs stades de l'évaluation de la sécurité chimique.

On fait appel à des modèles mathématiques pour simuler la dynamique du partage, de la diffusion, du métabolisme d'autres processus qui interviennent dans l'absorption percutanée, ce qui peut permettre de prédire dans quelle proportion et à quelle vitesse une substance chimique donnée va pénétrer à travers le revêtement cutané. Ces modèles mathématiques sont d'une importance primordiale pour établir la relation qui lie le coefficient de perméabilité et les données de flux fournies par l'expérimentation en régime stationnaire (c'est-à-dire à dose infinie) aux estimations de l'absorption en présence de doses finies qui sont plus représentatives de l'exposition professionnelle (c'est-à-dire en régime non stationnaire).

Lorsqu'on procède à l'évaluation du risque, l'estimation initiale de l'absorption percutanée est habituellement obtenue en opérant en plusieurs stades, la marge de sécurité maximale étant définie par le cas le plus critique et des estimations plus élaborées permettant une meilleure approximation de la marge réelle. Dans un premier temps, on suppose donc que l'absorption est de 100 % en l'absence de toute donnée. On procède ensuite à une deuxième évaluation plus réaliste de l'absorption percutanée en prenant en compte les propriétés physico-chimiques de la substance étudiée et de son véhicule. La troisième stade comporte la prise en considération de toute donnée expérimentale sur l'absorption percutanée tirée de tests in vitro ou in vivo. Si, à l'issue de ces trois étapes, le calcul montre que le risque est inacceptable, le meilleur moyen d'en affiner l'évaluation consiste à s'appuyer sur les valeurs effectives de l'exposition.

Au cours des dernières années, il y a eu, pour une part sous l'influence de la réglementation, un certain nombre d'initiatives en vue de faire progresser plus rapidement l'harmonisation au niveau international des méthodes et des protocoles expérimentaux. Ces initiatives ont abouti en 2004 à la publication par l'OCDE de lignes directrices expérimentales applicables aux études sur l'absorption percutanée. Cette coopération internationale se traduit par un certain nombre de projets tels qu'une étude internationale de validation à laquelle participent 18 laboratoires, le projet européen EDETOX (*European Evaluations and Predictions of Dermal Absorption of Toxic Chemicals*), ainsi que divers autres projets subventionnés par l'industrie ou encore des conférences telles que la conférence intitulée *Perspectives in Percutaneous Penetration* (précédemment intitulée *Prediction of Percutaneous Penetration* ou PPP) ou les *Gordon Research Conferences.* Les données existantes au sujet du flux transcutané et du coefficient d'absorption ont été recueillies dans des bases de données et analysées. On a également progressé dans l'élaboration de RQSA permettant de relier la pénétration transcutanée aux propriétés physico-chimiques des substances chimiques. On parvient ainsi à prédire de mieux en mieux la pénétration transcutanée d'un grand nombre de produits chimiques. Ces développements peuvent vraisemblablement contribuer à réduire l'expérimentation humaine et animale des produits chimiques qui est coûteuse et exigeante sur le plan éthique.

Malgré les succès obtenus jusqu'ici dans l'harmonisation interdisciplinaire au niveau international, des améliorations peuvent encore être apportées sur un certain nombre de points qui sont encore en discussion. Il s'agit notamment du degré de variation intralaboratoire et interlaboratoires des résultats d'études in vivo et in vitro, de l'acceptation des RQSP, de l'effet de réservoir des substances chimiques dans la couche cornée et de son interprétation pour l'évaluation du risque, de l'intérêt des mesures de l'absorption percutanée eu égard aux données demandées par ceux qui sont chargés de l'évaluation du risque et enfin de l'utilisation du test d'intégrité de la barrière cutanée pour évaluer la fonction de protection de la peau. Parmi les autres points à envisager figurent la valeur de l'absorption percutanée dans les populations sensibles, la nécessité d'harmoniser le système de notation cutanée et l'absorption percutanée des nanoparticules.

Le Groupe de travail a formulé des recommandations sur les points suivants : intérêt d'utiliser des échantillons de peau humaine plutôt que de peau animale; conception des études et harmonisation de la méthodologie; corrélation entre les données in vivo et in vitro et élaboration de modèles prédictifs fiables; incitation à soutenir, gérer et actualiser les bases de données; poursuite de l'évaluation des RQSA aux fins de l'évaluation du risque et préparation d'un guide en vue de leur utilisation.

RESUMEN

Absorción cutánea (percutánea, a través de la piel) es un término general que describe el transporte de sustancias químicas desde la superficie externa de la piel a su interior y a la circulación sistémica. El presente documento de la serie de Criterios de Salud Ambiental contiene un panorama general de la absorción cutánea y su aplicación a la evaluación del riesgo de las sustancias químicas. Además, se exponen y examinan temas actuales de interés en esta esfera. La absorción cutánea se puede producir a partir de la exposición de la piel a productos químicos, cosméticos y farmacéuticos en el trabajo, en el medio ambiente o en el consumo.

La piel es un órgano complejo y una membrana viva. Tiene funciones de protección, de regulación de la temperatura corporal y la pérdida de agua y de defensa y reparación. Se compone de una región externa, la epidermis, y una región interna, la dermis. La epidermis está formada por varias capas de células, la más externa de las cuales, el estrato córneo o capa córnea, funciona como barrera principal para la entrada de sustancias químicas extrañas. La epidermis viable puede metabolizar las sustancias químicas que pasan a través del sustrato córneo. La dermis proporciona apoyo fisiológico a la epidermis no vascular y en ella se localizan los vasos sanguíneos, los nervios sensoriales y los vasos linfáticos cutáneos. La piel contiene también otros apéndices, como los folículos pilosos, las glándulas sudoríparas y las glándulas sebáceas, cuya formación tiene lugar en la dermis subpapilar.

En la medición de la permeabilidad cutánea hay una variabilidad considerable. Puede haber diferencias importantes en la permeabilidad entre especies. Es poco lo que se conoce acerca de la variación debida a la edad, aunque la estructura de la piel cambia con el tiempo; sin embargo, la condición sexual o étnica no parece ser fuente de variación de la permeabilidad. La absorción percutánea depende asimismo del lugar anatómico, del estado de la piel y de su hidratación.

Los factores que influyen en la absorción percutánea a través de la piel son los siguientes: 1) propiedades fisicoquímicas del compuesto de prueba; 2) propiedades fisicoquímicas y de otro tipo del vehículo en el que está disuelto dicho compuesto; 3) interacciones entre este compuesto o el vehículo y la piel; 4) propiedades y metabolismo de la piel; y 5) factores inherentes al sistema de prueba utilizado para la medición, por ejemplo la dosis y el volumen de la sustancia de prueba, la oclusión o no de la zona de prueba, la utilización de sistemas de prueba *in vitro* o *in vivo* y la duración de la exposición.

Se han elaborado ecuaciones y modelos teóricos para describir el transporte de una sustancia química por difusión a través de la piel. Los principales parámetros evaluados en los experimentos *in vitro* son normalmente el flujo estacionario (J_{ss}) y el coeficiente de permeabilidad (K_p), en los cuales la concentración de la sustancia penetrante en la solución donante se mantiene en condiciones de dosificación (infinita) constante. Ahora se reconoce que la estimación del flujo máximo, el tiempo necesario para alcanzar el flujo máximo, el tiempo de demora, las cantidades residuales (reservorio) retenidas en el estrato córneo y el balance de masa en condiciones de aplicación "reales" son de importancia capital para las estimaciones de la exposición.

La medición del metabolismo de una sustancia química en contacto con la piel puede ser importante en las evaluaciones tanto de la eficacia como de la inocuidad. Algunas sustancias químicas se pueden metabolizar de manera significativa durante la absorción cutánea, lo que podría dar lugar a la formación de metabolitos inactivos o activos. Por consiguiente, la medición de este metabolismo puede ser importante en una evaluación apropiada de la inocuidad. Se ha demostrado que sustancias químicas tóxicas como el benzo[α]pireno se activan en la piel, mientras que otras pueden sufrir reacciones de hidrólisis y/o conjugación, con la consiguiente disminución de la disponibilidad de esas sustancias por el organismo. En general se puede mantener la viabilidad de la piel en una celda de difusión *in vitro* utilizando piel fresca y un tampón fisiológico. Se recomienda verificar esta viabilidad mediante la medición de la actividad de las enzimas metabólicas correspondientes.

La mayor parte de las propiedades de permeabilidad del estrato córneo se mantienen inalteradas después de su extracción del organismo. Así pues, existe una buena correlación entre las mediciones obtenidas en experimentos de difusión cutánea tanto *in vivo* como *in vitro* utilizando las mismas sustancias químicas (por lo menos para los compuestos hidrofílicos). Los experimentos *in vitro* son un sistema sustitutivo adecuado de los estudios *in vivo* y ofrecen varias ventajas sobre los experimentos con animales enteros o voluntarios humanos. Con los métodos *in vivo* se mide la difusión de las sustancias químicas hacia el interior de la piel y a través de ella hasta alcanzar un reservorio fluido y se puede utilizar piel no viable para medir sólo la difusión o piel fresca metabólicamente activa para medir al mismo tiempo la difusión y el metabolismo cutáneo. La Directriz 428 de Prueba de la Organización de Cooperación y Desarrollo Económicos (OCDE) alienta la armonización de la metodología. Otros factores experimentales que afectan a la absorción cutánea *in vitro*, además de los ya mencionados, son el grosor de la muestra de piel, las variaciones de temperatura en el sistema de prueba y la composición del fluido receptor. Se pueden utilizar celdas de difusión *in vitro* estáticas o de flujo continuo. Otras técnicas que requieren un ulterior perfeccionamiento son la extracción con tiras adhesivas (*tape stripping*) y la utilización de piel artificial o reconstituida.

Los métodos *in vivo* permiten determinar el grado de absorción cutánea, así como sistémica, de la sustancia de prueba. La ventaja principal de realizar un estudio *in vivo* en lugar de *in vitro* es que se utiliza un sistema intacto desde el punto de vista fisiológico y metabólico. Se realizan estudios de penetración cutánea *in vivo* en animales de laboratorio, normalmente roedores, y en voluntarios humanos. Estos últimos se han utilizado ampliamente para productos farmacéuticos de aplicación humana y en menor medida para otras sustancias químicas. El nivel máximo de garantía se obtiene mediante estudios *in vivo* con personas. La realización de cualquier estudio *in vivo* conlleva cuestiones éticas. La principal desventaja de utilizar animales de laboratorio es que tienen una permeabilidad cutánea y una disposición sistémica diferentes en comparación con las personas.

Los resultados de los estudios realizados con voluntarios humanos han puesto de manifiesto que la exposición ocupacional a líquidos (como disolventes) puede dar lugar a una absorción cutánea considerable. La absorción cutánea a partir de vapores puede contribuir de manera importante a la total de algunas sustancias volátiles, como los éteres de glicol.

Cada vez se presentan más estudios de absorción cutánea *in vitro* con fines de registro de sustancias químicas industriales, cosméticos y productos de protección de los cultivos. Se han publicado numerosos estudios en los que se comparan los resultados obtenidos *in vitro* e *in vivo* con animales de laboratorio y con personas. Los estudios *in vitro* realizados de manera adecuada siguiendo las directrices de prueba de la OCDE han puesto de manifiesto que los métodos *in vitro* pueden proporcionar una buena predicción de la absorción cutánea *in vivo*.

Durante decenios se ha obtenido información abundante sobre la penetración percutánea de un gran número de sustancias químicas, plaguicidas, cosméticos y productos farmacéuticos. Los estudios han incluido experimentos con voluntarios humanos, estudios *in vivo* con modelos animales, estudios *in vitro* con piel extraída por ejemplo de personas, roedores, cerdos y cobayas, y más recientemente estudios *in vitro* con piel sintética.

Durante los 50 últimos años se han realizado numerosos intentos de predecir la velocidad y el grado de la absorción cutánea, para de esta manera reducir la necesidad de realizar pruebas *in vitro* e *in vivo*. Esta necesidad es incluso mayor en respuesta a las crecientes dificultades éticas con respecto a la realización de experimentos con personas y animales de laboratorio, así como a las consideraciones económicas y temporales impuestas por la legislación, sobre todo con respecto a la evaluación del riesgo de las sustancias químicas industriales. La relación cuantitativa entre la estructura y la permeabilidad es una relación derivada estadísticamente entre el flujo estacionario de un compuesto y diversos descriptores fisicoquímicos y/o propiedades estructurales de la molécula. En las consideraciones relativas a la eficacia y la inocuidad también se reconoce la relación cuantitativa entre la estructura y la actividad en relación con la irritación, la sensibilización cutánea, el metabolismo, los efectos químicos y la eliminación. Por consiguiente, este tipo de relación interviene en varios niveles de la inocuidad química.

Se han utilizado modelos matemáticos para simular la dinámica de la distribución, difusión, metabolismo y otros procesos que intervienen en la absorción cutánea y pueden conducir a la predicción del grado y la velocidad de la permeación química a través de la piel. La creación de modelos matemáticos desempeña una función esencial en la vinculación del coeficiente de permeabilidad y los datos relativos al flujo obtenidos en pruebas realizadas en condiciones estacionarias (es decir, dosis infinita) con la estimación de la absorción para las aplicaciones de dosis finitas que son más habituales en la exposición ocupacional (es decir, condiciones no estacionarias).

En la evaluación del riesgo, la estimación inicial de la absorción cutánea se suele obtener mediante la utilización de un método estratificado, en el que el mayor margen de inocuidad se define por el caso peor y las estimaciones más ajustadas definen mejor el margen real. Por consiguiente, como primer paso se supone que la absorción es del 100% cuando no se dispone de datos. En segundo lugar se proporciona un estimación más realista del grado de absorción cutánea mediante un análisis de las propiedades fisicoquímicas de la sustancia química y del vehículo. En tercer lugar se realiza un estudio de todos los datos experimentales de absorción cutánea *in vitro* e *in vivo*. Si al final de estas etapas se calcula un riesgo inaceptable, la mejor manera de ajustar la evaluación del riesgo es mediante los datos de exposición real.

En los últimos años, debido en parte a presiones normativas, ha habido varias iniciativas para acelerar los progresos en la armonización internacional de la metodología y los protocolos, que culminaron con la publicación en 2004 de las directrices de prueba de la OCDE para los estudios de absorción cutánea. Esta colaboración internacional incluye proyectos tales como un estudio de validación internacional con la participación de 18 laboratorios, el proyecto de evaluaciones europeas y predicciones de la absorción cutánea de sustancias químicas tóxicas (EDETOX) y proyectos patrocinados por la industria, así como conferencias, por ejemplo sobre las Perspectivas en la penetración percutánea (anteriormente, Predicción de la penetración percutánea, o PPP) y las "Gordon Research Conferences". Los datos disponibles sobre los flujos cutáneos y los coeficientes de permeabilidad se han recogido en bases de datos y se han analizado. Se ha avanzado en el perfeccionamiento ulterior de las relaciones cuantitativas entre la estructura y la actividad que vinculan los datos de permeación con las propiedades fisicoquímicas de las sustancias químicas. Por consiguiente, cada vez son mayores las posibilidades de predecir de manera más fidedigna los datos de penetración para un gran número de sustancias químicas. Un posible resultado es la reducción de las pruebas que son costosas y exigentes desde el punto de vista ético de las sustancias químicas utilizando animales de laboratorio y personas.

A pesar del éxito alcanzado hasta ahora en la armonización internacional interdisciplinaria, hay algunos aspectos susceptibles de mejora y que siguen siendo objeto de debate. Son el grado de variación en los estudios *in vitro* e *in vivo* dentro de un laboratorio y entre laboratorios; la aceptación de la relación cuantitativa entre la estructura y la permeabilidad; el efecto de reservorio de las sustancias químicas en el estrato córneo y su interpretación en la evaluación del riesgo; la pertinencia de las mediciones de la absorción cutánea para los datos que necesitan los evaluadores del riesgo; y la utilización de la prueba de integridad de la barrera para la función protectora de la piel. Otros temas que se pueden examinar son la absorción cutánea en poblaciones susceptibles, la necesidad de armonizar la anotación cutánea y la absorción cutánea de nanopartículas.

El Grupo de Trabajo formula recomendaciones sobre los beneficios de la utilización de la piel humana en comparación con la piel de animales de laboratorio; la formulación del estudio y la armonización de la metodología; la correlación de los datos obtenidos *in vitro* e *in vivo* y la creación de modelos de predicción fidedignos; el fomento del apoyo, el mantenimiento y la actualización de las bases de datos; y la promoción de la evaluación de la relación cuantitativa entre la estructura y la permeabilidad con fines de evaluación del riesgo y la preparación de orientaciones sobre su utilización.

www.ingramcontent.com/pod-product-compliance
Ingram Content Group UK Ltd.
Pitfield, Milton Keynes, MK11 3LW, UK
UKHW021313180426
11947UKWH00015B/1191

9 789241 572354